EPIDEMIC

EPIDEMIC

The Past, Present and Future
of the Diseases that Made Us

Dr Robert Baker

First published in 2007 by Vision Paperbacks,
a division of Satin Publications Ltd
101 Southwark Street
London SE1 0JF
UK
info@visionpaperbacks.co.uk
www.visionpaperbacks.co.uk
Publisher: Sheena Dewan

A catalogue record for this book is available
from the British Library.

978-1-905745-08-1

2 4 6 8 10 9 7 5 3 1

Cover photo: Getty Images/3D4Medical.com
Cover and text design by ok?design
Printed and bound in the UK by
Mackays of Chatham Ltd, Chatham, Kent

CONTENTS

ACKNOWLEDGEMENTS

It is only right that I acknowledge the contribution of various people who helped bring this book about. I am grateful to my agent, Charlotte Howard, for introducing me to the publishers. Thank you to Charlotte Cole for commissioning it.

Much of my understanding of the science of microbiology was derived from my time at King's College Hospital, London, while working with Drs John Philpot-Howard, Jim Wade, Ian Eltringham and Amanda Fife. Similarly Bob Wall and Rob Davidson at Northwick Park Hospital, and Armine Sefton at Bart's and the London were inspirational. I am indebted to all of them for demonstrating how fascinating and important the science of microbiology can be. I am also hugely grateful to the great Professor Brian Gazzard of the Chelsea and Westminster Hospital for triggering a lasting interest in human immuno-deficiency virus (HIV) medicine.

I would like to thank my great friends Alfie Kaye, Edward

ACKNOWLEDGEMENTS

Bruce and Rafe Elliot for stimulating and enlivening debate while I was working on the book. It is dedicated to my wife and family, particularly my eldest son Matthew – yes, it's finished now, we can go outside and play football.

INTRODUCTION

One for the slaughter

Private Tommy Jones of the Royal Sussex Regiment woke up feeling fine and set about his morning duties. It was a rainy November morning; parade had been called off. Feeding the pigs was a welcome relief from the relentless bayonet practice, parade ground drill and lectures on gas attacks, typhus and trench fever from brutal old hands that filled the days. Tommy was stationed at the infamous Bull Ring training camp at Etaples. He had been a farm labourer in civilian life and enjoyed working with animals; he liked tipping the big buckets of swill to the eager, untidy beasts. This morning as usual he was followed by gulls who competed for the easy pickings on his cart. A few days ago he had bought a goose from a local farmer; he had plucked and drawn it himself. He and his mates had feasted happily that night. He knew it was only a matter of time before he was sent up the line;

he tried not to think about the trainload of muddy, bloodstained and pale casualties, some already dead, pulling in to Boulogne when he disembarked just three weeks earlier. Me and the pigs, he thought; both of us have a date with the butcher. He was more accurate than he could know.

Immediately after dinner he began to feel a little odd, as he told Captain Travers, the medical officer. He wondered if it was the afternoon's training drill, where he had had to run through a gas-filled shed. Maybe it was the compulsory typhoid vaccination that all his pals had hated so much; many of them had been ill but most had recovered. The MO curtly dismissed his claim about the vaccine; he wasn't standing for any barrack-room backchat. Jones' head ached furiously. He felt hot and sweaty, and his back and calves felt like he had done a week's square bashing in an hour.

Tommy never made it to his appointment with the trenches. He died the next day: a horrible death, where his breathing became increasingly difficult and ultimately he drowned in his own lung fluids. The skin around his mouth, fingers and ears turned a dusky blue. He died of acute pneumonia, caused by the influenza virus. He had contracted it from the goose.

The date was 1916. Within three years 50 million or more were to be dead from the same disease, the majority of them in 1918. More than smallpox, more than the Black Death, more even than the Great War itself. Astonishingly, this disease killed more soldiers on both sides than bullets, bombs or gas. It might even have shortened the war.

We do not know that Tommy existed, but many like him did: his story is based on historical events and scientific plausibility.

Nobody knows for certain where the first cases of H1N1 influenza, known as the Spanish Lady, arose. However, it is known that there were multiple cases of troops dying from an unexplained disease which caused them to turn blue (known as heliotrope cyanosis by contemporary pathologists) in the British Army's Bull Ring training camp at Etaples from the winter of 1916 onwards. This was one of the main holding and training camps for troops heading for the slaughter of the Western Front. Up to 100,000 soldiers were encamped there at any one time.

Other authorities claim that the first cases arose in China, or in a military camp in Kansas in the United States in 1918, but the Bull Ring disease predates both by two years, so if it was H1N1, it is the earliest known occurrence of it. The disease became known as 'Spanish' probably because Spain had no censorship in those years. What has become clear is that the virus originated in birds, and mutated possibly via pigs, to spread between humans. There were pigs kept for fodder at the Bull Ring, and soldiers were known to have bought poultry from local farmers, so the conditions were right for Spanish flu to take hold. Many soldiers at the time incorrectly blamed the typhoid vaccine. The mass demobilisation of troops and their subsequent return home could then, if the hypothesis is correct, have transmitted the disease across the globe. If you were going to design a method of spreading an epidemic to the world, you could not do better than this.

Old threats, new threats

Is it going to happen again? Not so many years ago a book about epidemics would probably have been classified as history.

That might have made its contents seem harmless and sterile. It is only the present and the future that can hold any real menace. The past is not only a foreign country, it is a safe country to visit. Most of the threats and dangers of that past have been mapped out, and we can simply and safely observe them. However, this foreign country may have decided to mobilise its armies and attempt an invasion. Epidemics no longer represent a theoretical, distant, emasculated hazard. As the 21st century progresses, their formidable power imperils us once again, and this book is in part about that increasing threat. It will examine the nature of the life-forms that put us individually and collectively in jeopardy, their biology, how they are transmitted, why they are coming back and how they make us ill. Some of the effects of our constant exposure to both hostile and pacific elements in the natural world are far from obvious. Even less obvious are the consequences of humankind's efforts to control and avoid them, sometimes to our disadvantage, as we shall see.

Although many of the infectious hazards we face seem new, and indeed some are new, we need to interpret them in the context of what has gone before. It is easy to forget to what an extent infectious diseases threatened humankind in the past. 'New' infectious diseases often turn out not to be so new after all, or may be extensions of existing epidemics. For instance, when Willy Burgdorfer, an eminent specialist in the typhus-causing bacteria called rickettsiae, began to investigate the outbreak of a new form of arthritis that afflicted children in Old Lyme, Connecticut in 1976, he found that descriptions of an identical illness could be found in literature from the previous century. And the epidemic that caused profuse watery diarrhoea and sometimes even death in Bangladesh in 1971, during the civil war and following a tidal wave, was actually part of a much wider existing cholera epidemic known as El Tor. Some other aspects of our current plight are also a legacy of the past. It is patently obvious that we cannot really understand the emergence of microbes that are resistant to drugs without considering the mistakes of the past and the way in which living organisms have evolved.

In addition, our methods of tackling epidemics are based on long-standing principles that have been historically tried and tested. The concept of containment and quarantine for infectious illness was accepted – and effective – long before the nature of the life-forms that cause disease was established. We do have allies in our foreign country.

This book

Epidemic divides up the main epidemics by the nature of the microbes that cause them – viruses, bacteria, parasites, fungi, yeasts and those peculiar apparently non-living agents of disease, prions. I shall use this structure, together with brief case histories (with identities disguised to protect the victims), to highlight how the varying nature of the life-forms with which we share our planet dictates the manner in which they cause illness.

This might give the slightly misleading impression that fungi and yeasts, for example, are as important as a cause of epidemics as viruses and bacteria. While it is actually true that a yeast causes one of the world's most common sexually transmitted diseases, a fact that even most doctors find surprising, generally fungi and yeasts rarely cause epidemics. I am not a soothsayer, and cannot promise that this will always be so. For all I know there is a highly transmissible fungus lurking in a cave somewhere, awaiting its moment to wreak havoc on humans. There is already one such fungus, *Histoplasma capsulatum*, which skulks in bat caves and occasionally causes fatal disease even in healthy people, in places including California's aptly named Death Valley. I shall also examine the reasons that I think more widespread outbreaks of fungal illness are unlikely, however.

This book has a deeper theme, and an essential premise. That premise is that humankind is epidemics. This slightly ungrammatical statement contains the essential argument on which the book is constructed. Put more bluntly, humanity is infectious diseases. This applies, in some sense, to all aspects of human biology, behaviour, culture, history and technology. If the book is successful in its aims, it will cause you to completely reconsider what we are, what we are made from, how we got here and where we are going.

The human disease

Infectious disease has moulded us even at the most obvious and superficial level. Consider the human face: with a little imagination, every aspect of its appearance may be considered to be concerned with the prevention of infectious disease. Take, for instance, the structure of the eyes. This is of course determined by the properties of light, but their physical appearance has been dictated by something else. They are shiny, because you secrete tears which wash them every time you blink. These tears contain chemicals which prevent your eyes from becoming infected. The shape of the visible eye is determined by the lids. The lids cover the eyes to prevent them from drying out and becoming infected, and to wash the disinfecting material over their surface. Your lips are red, because they are covered in a specialised kind of skin that is more flexible and more able to regenerate than the tougher skin of your cheeks and the rest of your body. Without this lip tissue your mouth would tear and become infected. The skin of your face will be very slightly greasy, especially if you have not washed for a while. Contained within the grease are substances that both combat infection and permit harmless bacteria to inhabit your skin as friendly, protective passengers. I could continue this list almost indefinitely: your hair, teeth, ears, all have evolved in part to protect you from infection.

The same is true of humanity collectively. In its most obvious form there is no doubt that current human behaviour represents a kind of epidemic of its own, with the victim being our own planet. Thomas Malthus predicted that human population would be limited by competition for food. On the evidence so far, he was wrong; the massive population growth since Malthus' time has been readily, if inequitably, sustained by the food supplies of our world. Even now it is not lack of food, but our excessive production of waste products, in the form of gases like carbon dioxide, that is currently believed to threaten our welfare. Happily for the sake of my argument, but unhappily for the planet, we face exactly the same problem as rapidly multiplying colonies of bacteria: we are risking our future by poisoning ourselves with our own exhausts. There is symmetry in this conclusion, in that the early conditions for life to develop were almost certainly made possible by the earliest life-forms consuming gases that were too toxic to support life, and emitting oxygen. Those life-forms resembled bacteria more than anything else. They may even prove our salvation.

This book takes the theory a stage further by arguing that epidemics of infectious disease best explain how humanity came about. It is thus a self-centred book, unapologetically centred around the universe of my own experience and knowledge as a microbiologist. If I were an evolutionary biologist, I might reasonably advance the claim that Darwinian evolution most accurately answers the question of who we are and how we arose. If I were a molecular biologist, I might point to the precise constellations and sequences of base pairs in the DNA helix, and claim they were the key to life, the universe and everything. A biochemist would probably advance the premise that biochemical processes were at the heart of all existence; without the various pathways of sugar, oxygen and phosphate metabolism there could be no life. For my purposes all of these apparently conflicting hypotheses are simultaneously true. It is the mark of advanced minds like yours and mine that they can accept paradox. Besides, as we shall explore, all things are connected.

But there are many other ways in which the statement that humankind is epidemics can be interpreted, and they will be explored in these pages. Epidemics of infectious diseases have shaped our past and our destiny. Many of the ways in which they have done so are obvious. Wars have been won and lost as a consequence of epidemics. The pandemic of influenza may have hastened the 1918 armistice. Cortes' victory over the Aztecs relied as much upon the slaughter of the native population by smallpox and measles as it did upon military victory. On at least one occasion conquest was deliberately achieved by the release of infectious agents like smallpox to a population under siege. To earlier generations, some parts of the world were uninhabitable because of the constant threat of diseases like malaria and sleeping sickness.

Major historical figures have suffered from epidemic infectious diseases, and the course of history has been altered as a result. A fine example is Oliver Cromwell, who not only died young, probably from malaria, but whose bigotry and anti-Catholicism caused a global epidemic of lethal yellow fever, which lasted for at least two centuries.

Although these diseases are now at least partly controllable, epidemics have as much geopolitical impact today as they ever did. Few could doubt that epidemics of bubonic plague altered the social and economic structure of Europe forever. That sort of process is being repeated in countries across the globe today, as the HIV/AIDS epidemic wreaks its terrible toll. Trends in longevity have been reduced and improvements in economic prosperity almost destroyed in some nations by the burden of a single viral illness. Countries where the prevalence of HIV approaches 50 per cent, and where there is not the money or the infrastructure to confront and treat the disease, will have their future defined by this epidemic.

So epidemic infectious diseases have made us what we are, and in a deeper sense we even *are* infectious diseases. We shall examine that peculiar statement in detail in Chapter 2, but perhaps I need to explain it briefly here. Close analysis of the structure of human and animal cells reveals something of an anomaly. Not all the contents of our cells 'belong' to us. There are constituents that clearly have more in common with ancient bacteria and newer viruses than they do with humans or animals. Specifically, cell components called mitochondria are almost certainly purple sulphur bacteria of the sort found in geothermal vents at the floors of the oceans. They almost certainly came to be within our cells because of an antediluvian 'epidemic' which afflicted our primordial ancestors. Primitive single-celled amoeba-like structures became infected by bacteria, and we are still in a sense infected by them now.

Nor does it stop there. When we examine the very first origins of life itself, the process may have had much in common with an infectious, epidemic process. How did the leap from inert, inorganic and organic molecules to life happen? One very reasonable explanation involves a process of spontaneous self-assembly of naturally occurring substances. (This is discussed at more length in Chapter 1, on viruses.) One hypothesis is that the earliest near-life forms resembled viruses. They were believed to be short stretches of RNA, rather like basic viruses. These brief, initially random, compilations of molecules would have been able to interact with other similar forms, and 'infect' neighbouring sequences, perhaps creating an organism with increased complexity and function. All life, including that of humans, might have come to exist as a result of such 'infections', and it can be no surprise that infections still form much of the substance of our existence.

It's in our genes

An analysis of human genes reveals that there are large sequences of DNA that unquestionably arose from unexpected sources. Examining patterns of DNA sequences gives clear clues to their origins; put simply not all genes seem to have arisen by simple evolution. The common view is that genes show the pattern they do because of a process of natural selection. Organisms with successful characteristics are more likely to reproduce, so these characteristics are selectively passed from one generation to another. In fact evolution has been far more inclusive. It now appears that a very large proportion of our genes arose in other life forms, and 'infected' us. These are the so-called mobile genetic elements, and many are of viral or bacterial origin. Sometimes I amuse myself by asking medical students how many of their genes come from this source. Occasionally someone will make a wild guess of 100 per cent, but most sensible people would probably put the figure much lower. Even so; you may be surprised to discover that the answer is 45 per cent.

Some of these elements are of particular importance, and the subject of intense, cutting-edge research. These are known as human endogenous retroviruses (HERVs). The Human Genome Project was completed in 2003. It has identified all the 20,000–25,000 genes in human DNA. Since that project was finished, it has even been possible to measure the proportion of the genes in our chromosomes that came from these viruses. The best available figure is astonishing: it amounts to a staggering 8 per cent of our DNA.

In other words, what we have learnt about evolutionary history through the study of our genes has made it clear that we have acquired genes, whether we use them or not, through the invasion of our cells by viruses. Almost certainly we owe much of our complexity to the fact that we acquired genes from these viruses. Some hypothesise that the great difference between humans and other animals – the property of self-awareness – arose through viral infection. We shall briefly discuss this later in the book. Whether that is true or not, the activity of these viral genes is a subject of considerable interest.

Probably the most important thing we have learnt to date is that these viral incorporations are not random. They are carried forward in more or less the same form from one generation to the next, and are shared by all humans. Even if we do not know what their function is now, it seems likely as a result that at least at some point in our evolutionary history, they had a useful function, and that is why they were preserved. There is also accumulating evidence that they may be responsible for some cancers and auto-immune diseases. This science is in its infancy and has not produced absolutely conclusive evidence. Nevertheless the point remains valid – in a very real physical and genetic sense, we are epidemics.

Immunity and evolution

Infectious epidemics have also shaped our evolution by other, more conventional means. At one extreme this might mean straightforward Darwinian selection whereby all individuals who lack protection from an epidemic might die, with a smaller proportion who carry the necessary protective gene left to repopulate. However, human evolution may operate more subtly and with greater complexity. Infectious epidemics have provided a constant evolutionary challenge which we as a species have constantly had to meet.

Some scientists refer to this as the 'Red Queen' hypothesis, after the character in Lewis Carroll's *Alice in Wonderland* who had to run faster and faster in order to remain in the same place. Our immunity has, without doubt, evolved in response to the challenge of epidemics. Without infection there would be little point in even having an immune system.

We can pursue this argument a stage further. As understanding of science evolves, it is becoming clear that body 'systems' do not operate in isolation. The hormones of the endocrine system interact with the immune system in ways of enormous sophistication; indeed, in some senses there is very little difference between a classical hormone like insulin and the chemical messengers of immunity. Our nervous systems and brains are equally closely involved with combating infection. Thus a species of organism that struggles with infectious epidemics will increase in complexity in all its body systems, including hormones, the brain and the nervous system.

We could, of course, argue that all animals (and indeed plants) must meet the challenge of infection; why should we not apply the same arguments to them? The answer is that of course we can. Plants, animals and other life-forms owe their essence as much to the infections they encounter as we human beings do. Powerful further evidence for the fact that other life-forms contend with infectious disease is contained in the famous story of Fleming's observation of penicillin, and the subsequent almost immediate emergence of resistance to that chemical.

Penicillin is a drug that attacks bacteria. It was initially obtained from, and produced by, a mould. Fleming noticed that some strains of bacteria were able to produce enzymes that inactivated the penicillin molecule as soon as they encountered it. They did this more rapidly than it might have been predicted from evolutionary processes, which should have required many generations of evolution before being able to work out this trick. The explanation for this is that the mould and the bacteria had met before. The enzymes already existed in nature, as a consequence of previous struggles between them.

The bulk of the antibiotic compounds now in common use were essentially derived from the same source; that is, they are natural products of existing organisms. There is no doubt that such antibiotics have altered the course of human history for the better. Once-dreaded scourges such as syphilis – the Great Pox, as our ancestors knew it – have practically been vanquished, and by straightforward penicillin at that. Effective treatments for battle wounds unquestionably affected the outcome of the Second World War; up until at least the American Civil War the number of soldiers unfit for combat through infectious illness such as diarrhoea at least equalled the number wounded or killed on the battlefield.

Like us, plants and other animals share some odd properties that do not, at first sight, appear to have arisen from conventional evolutionary processes. Why do we have half of our genes in common with bananas? Why do peas, for example, carry the genes that encode haemoglobin, the molecule that carries oxygen in animal blood? The explanation may be that peas evolved from organisms that required haemoglobin. Another explanation is that peas, bananas and humans became infected by viruses carrying common genes.

So if plants and other animals also owe their essential nature to infection, why do I emphasise the point to the extreme in humans? The straightforward answer to this question is that simpler organisms are susceptible to a narrower range of infections. If a plant is composed of many copies of near-identical cells, then the target range for infecting organisms will be narrower. Many infections rely on some variety of specific interaction between the infectious agent and receptors on the host's cell; if the receptor is absent, the infection cannot occur. Some species of plant are targeted by a single, specific strain of virus. Whether the ultimate variety of infections to which a species is susceptible is a consequence of that organism's complexity or a cause of it is open to debate. However, I shall argue that it is a cause, purely on the basis of empirical evidence.

Of course it is in our interests, and within our abilities, to characterise the infections that the human flesh is heir to. Therefore we know more about human diseases than we do about those that affect any other species. However, even given the bias inherent in that state of affairs, it remains true that humans are susceptible to more varieties of infection than any other organism with which we share the planet. That is a simple numerical fact. This is in part a reflection of the variety and complexity of different types of human cell, and the genetic variability within our species.

Now consider the evolutionary challenges which have decided that complexity. Most of the variables – climate, access to water and food, overcrowding, avoidance of predators – are limited in their possible consequences. Only one evolutionary challenge meets the necessary requirements that result in the extraordinary complexity of the human species, and that is infectious disease. More than any other animal, we are who we are because of them.

Trade-offs and complexity

Epidemics have shaped us in another way, and that is in our susceptibility to non-infectious disease. This may seem counter-intuitive, but there are multiple examples. We shall encounter them throughout the book, but the essence of the hypothesis is that resistance to epidemics sometimes comes at a cost. This is the well-established phenomenon called balanced polymor-phism, whereby disease-causing traits are inherited as a trade-off for disease resistance. As we shall also see, many non-infectious diseases like diabetes, allergies and cancers have clear causal links to epidemics of infections.

Not all of our encounters with epidemics have been to our detriment. Of particular interest here is the strange story of HIV resistance, which, we have discovered, is mediated through a mutant cell product called CCR5 delta-32. The delta-32 variant has been shown to be present in bronze-age skeletons. We only properly encountered HIV in the early 1980s. Why would a gene mutant that confers resistance to HIV have predated the onset of the disease itself by hundreds of years? We shall explore the reasons for this remarkable coincidence in Chapter 1.

Evolution and knowledge

There are those who argue that human evolution has moved on from simple transmission of genes through reproduction, into a more advanced and abstract sphere. The evolution of ideas in many respects mimics the evolution of species. The basic unit of information transfer – the equivalent of a gene in this abstract sphere – is called a meme, and the science of knowledge evolution is called memetics. It would not stretch the imagination too far to compare the collective insanity of, say, Nazism, to an outbreak of infectious disease with memes as the units of infection.

This 'super-evolution' has had a number of beneficial consequences for humankind in the context of epidemics. We have learnt from our past experience. We have been able to avoid or limit epidemics by conscious collective action, in a way that no other species can. No other animal practises quarantine in the way that humans have understood and adopted since ancient times. The importance of a supply of clean water and the controlled disposal of effluent in preventing the spread of disease have been understood for thousands of years. No matter how much we may admire them, even our closest and most evolved relatives in the animal kingdom are incapable of such strategies.

As humankind has advanced in knowledge, the struggle against epidemics has been at the very forefront of our development and progress. It has moved forward hand in hand with increasing industrial and technological sophistication. Indeed, many of the processes by which infections are identified arose through improved industrial technology. For example, the manufacture of synthetic dyes and precision milling of glass for microscopes have both been crucial in the science of microbiology, and both were the by-products of commercial industry. It may be stretching a point slightly to say that the highest achievements of our species have come in learning how to combat infectious diseases (especially as treatable diseases still kill so many), but these examples do illustrate the capacity for planned, altruistic cooperation which so distinguishes us from other animals. Almost by definition, we are tool-using animals. The fact that those tools might be Petri dishes, or sewers, or antibiotics, does not alter that.

Win some, fight more

The unintended consequences of all this technological development have been further epidemics. These are of the kind that define much of the experience of being a modern human. For example, we have seen an unexpected huge increase in the incidence of diseases such as allergies and asthma. One hypothesis (which we shall explore here) is that our modern addiction to soap and water has led to this epidemic. Although allergic diseases are not unknown among animals, they are far less common than among humans. Interestingly, such diseases are more common among domestic pets than wild animals, which may be for the same reason that modern humans seem to be more prone to them. Put simply, we are victims of our own cleverness. We and our pets, in our controlled and safe modern world, are no longer exposed to the infectious diseases with which we evolved. We are safer as a result, but we may have lost something important.

The relative triumph of the 19th and 20th centuries in tackling the dragging burden of constant epidemics, in large part through the application of science and technology, permitted the evolution of humankind into its current form. It is generally held (if disputed by some) that the fact that we managed to reduce the burden of disease allowed more children to survive into adulthood, and this in turn led to a massive increase in population.

Some of the other consequences of reduced susceptibility to epidemics might seem less obvious, but they may have been equally momentous. For example, mothers who were not diseased would have had healthier pregnancies, with reduced maternal and infant mortality. As an example, a chronic disease like tuberculosis would have compounded malnutrition. Infections of long duration may behave like cancers, and consume scarce nutrients. Such infections may also cause suppression of the appetite, with a consequent further reduction in the intake of food and vitamins. Mothers who suffered from both tuberculosis and malnutrition tended to have excessively narrow birth canals, and these would have more often resulted in the death of both mother and baby in childbirth. Reducing the incidence of tuberculosis would have broken this vicious circle.

This increasing population made greater demands of the new industries. The insatiable demand for new technologies during the industrial revolution was driven more by the suddenly huge number of individuals demanding clothing, food and transport than it was by a few brilliant individuals with a couple of new ideas.

We are now living with the consequences of that leap in population, fuelled as it was by technology and industry. Freedom from epidemics has allowed us to become, paradoxically, a more virulent epidemic of our own. I suggested early in this introduction that humankind has become an epidemic on the face of the planet, risking its own future by profligate emission of waste products. The price of our emergence from the shadow of infectious epidemics is being paid in the form of the 'carbon footprint' of the western way of life. This way of life has been exported, almost like an infectious disease, to the developing nations of the world, with inevitable consequences for the ecological future of our globe.

There are further consequences of this in the context of epidemic disease. It is increasingly clear that the climate of our world is changing, and many fear that the distribution of epidemic infectious diseases will alter as a consequence. The threat of diseases traditionally found in tropical zones, such as leishmaniasis or malaria, returning to northern Europe is more than just theoretical. Furthermore, the majority of 'new' infectious diseases such as Nipah virus, Hendra and even HIV have arisen from humans exploiting new ecological habitats for large-scale financial gain, or from encroachment into regions of low population density.

All good journeys end where they began, and so it is with us and epidemics. We arose from them, were moulded by them, nearly controlled them and now we are having to face them again. In part this is the result of emerging resistance to antibiotics, changing climate and disease patterns, and almost uncontrollable epidemics such as HIV/AIDS. Paradoxically, our near-escape from infections – at least in the West – makes us more vulnerable to their effects. When we live long enough to escape death from infection, we are more likely to die of cancer or auto-immune or heart disease. Both cancer and auto-immune diseases unquestionably have an infectious component. Heart disease may have one too, and each has a genetic component which may well have arisen from ancient viral infection. Furthermore, if the gloomiest predictions of those who warn us about global warming are correct, then our civilisation faces its greatest challenge of all. Civilisations in decline are particularly vulnerable to mass epidemics. As we began, so shall we end.

A choice of epidemics

Now I have outlined the basic premise of the book, it is time to consider which epidemics interest us the most. This is my 'hit parade' of top epidemics. Each of them is mentioned in the text, although not all are necessarily covered in great historical detail. They are introduced in order to illustrate a point about epidemics and their relationship with humans. This is not a complete list, and to make it into a round top ten (plus two) I have had to exclude some and cheat slightly by lumping some together.

It would be possible to argue for hours about which epidemics belong in any hit parade. For the purposes of this book the definition of an epidemic is an intuitive rather than an academic one. There is a difference, which I do not propose to explore. Most of these diseases appear in my list because of the sheer numbers who died or were affected. Some epidemic diseases were only rarely fatal, such as the recent increase in non-HIV sexually transmitted infections. The figures for some of the earlier historical epidemics are difficult to confirm, and should be taken as estimates. The cause of some of them can only be speculative, as contemporary science could not provide proof. Some other epidemics are discussed in the book because they contain revealing kernels of information about infections and us, but were not of the same scale; they do not appear in this list.

1 **The great influenza (Spanish flu)** epidemic of 1918–20. This killed approximately 50–100 million people (exact figures are unknown) in a very brief period, and had a particularly high mortality rate among young adults. This makes it the most lethal pandemic in known history. Should its mortality be repeated with our larger modern population of about 6 billion (compared with 1.8 billion in 1918) it would kill in excess of 300 million. This catastrophe is relatively fresh in human memory; there are even a few (if dwindling) survivors from the period. It is not hard to understand our current trepidation about influenza, especially as it is still responsible for an average of 36,000 deaths a year in the United States alone. Nor was this the first great influenza epidemic. The Asiatic (Russian) flu of 1889–90 killed at least

250,000 in Western Europe, and involved both North and South America. The peculiarities of this virus and its ability to transform itself make it probably our worst potential enemy. Many think we are not properly prepared for its inevitable reappearance.

2 **The Black Death** arose in the 14th century, with serial peaks of epidemics up until the 18th century, and sporadic outbreaks into the modern era. It is said to have killed 34 million people in Europe alone, with similar numbers in Asia. Africa and the Middle East were also affected, especially in the first epidemic of 1348–49. The global total during the 300 years of successive major epidemics was similar to that of the Spanish flu, but clearly over a much longer period. The generally held view is that these great plagues were caused by the bacterium *Yersinia pestis,* but there is continuing debate about whether a virus resembling Ebola was responsible; other diseases have also been suggested. The plague of Justinian of 541 AD may be included as part of the Black Death. It is thought to have killed 25 per cent of the population of the Mediterranean shore region.

3 **Malaria** is one of the foremost killers, in both the ancient and the modern world. A theoretically preventable disease, more or less eradicated in the West, it is responsible for 2.7 million deaths a year, a substantial

number being children – the World Health Organization (WHO) states that in the order of 2,800 children die of it each day. Many worry that global climate change will permit this scourge to return, even in Europe. It is already changing its distribution in some parts of the world.

4 The 'modern' epidemic of **sexually transmitted infections**, of which **HIV/AIDS** must be counted as the most dramatic and tragic. The exact date of its origin is debated, but the earliest known positive blood specimen dates from 1959. This modern plague really gathered pace in the early 1980s, since when the death toll has amounted to 26 million. Apart from the sheer numbers, this epidemic has transformed entire national economies, and some believe it threatens global security. Associated with this most disastrous of human events is the worldwide explosion of other sexually transmitted infections, including a dramatic increase in the numbers of young people with herpes, chlamydia and gonorrhoea, as well as other exotic sexually transmitted infections which occur in tropical countries which enhance HIV transmission. We are beginning to see some of these in Europe. Syphilis, then known as the Great Pox, appeared in Europe in the late 15th century, and was not truly controlled until penicillin became widely available in the 1940s. There has been a 1,000 per cent increase in new cases of syphilis in the United Kingdom since 1977.

5   **Cholera** is a bacterial disease spread in contaminated water and food. We are currently still in the seventh cholera pandemic, which began in 1961. The first arose in Calcutta in 1817, and involved the whole of India, China and southern Russia. The best records were kept by the British Army in India, which recorded 100,000 deaths. It was not confined to the military and nobody knows for certain how many died, but it is believed to extend into millions. Non-cholera diarrhoeal diseases are still a major cause of death in developing countries, killing between 1 and 2 million children under five every year.

6   **Smallpox** has been one of the great historical scourges, and during the Antonine plague of 165–180 AD it may have killed as many as 5 million. The West must accept both guilt and honour over this viral disease. On the one hand concerted effort by the WHO, largely funded by the developed nations, had eradicated the disease by 1977. On the other, there is no doubt that it caused catastrophe when introduced to the aboriginal populations of North and South America, in at least one case deliberately. Some believe there were something like 75 million people living in the Americas before Columbus, with about 12 million in North America. The 1900 US Census estimated the number of Native Americans to have collapsed to a mere 237,000. Of course not all of this decline can have been the result of smallpox, but as

we shall see, viruses like this one and measles, which also claimed many lives, behave very differently among people who have no history of exposure to the disease and encounter it at different ages.

As has been said above, Cortes' conquest of the Incas with a tiny force of soldiers was in no small part due to the diseases they brought with them, including smallpox and measles. Measles (which is of course distinct from smallpox) remains a major killer in the developing world, and was responsible for the depopulation of many parts of the world during the colonial expansion of European nations. It is a disease that has not gone away; there were an estimated 530,000 deaths in 2003. This figure is falling, from 873,000 in 1999, and the reason for that is absolutely cast-iron – vaccination. Scientific fact and conclusive evidence that the measles, mumps and rubella (MMR) vaccine is safe have proved inadequate for some to trust it, and as a result of varying take-up of the vaccine there have been troubling outbreaks in some European countries, notably Britain, Ireland and the Netherlands.

7   The same has been true of **poliomyelitis**, the cause of infant paralysis, and the first viral disease to be recorded in antiquity. When the global polio eradication campaign was launched in 1988, it was paralysing 1,000 children a day and killing many thousands; it has a mortality rate of 20–30 per cent. The 1916 polio

outbreak killed 6,000 in the United States alone. In 2003, fewer than 800 children were paralysed by the virus. This was the disease scheduled for eradication for 2005 by WHO, and it seemed within reach until there was a disastrous development, fuelled by conspiracy theorists and paranoid zealots. We will explore those events in Chapter 1.

8 **Typhus,** the bacterium carried by lice that killed its discoverer, Ricketts, is the disease of war and famine *par excellence.* It is impossible to estimate the total toll from *Rickettsia prowazekii,* but it may have been the agent of the Plague of Athens in 420 BC, according to David Durack, one of the world's foremost infectious disease physicians. The plague may have lost the Athenians the war against the Peloponnesian League, led by Sparta. Colossal mortality occurred during Napoleon's 1815 retreat from Moscow, the Irish potato famine and the First World War. Inhumanity in its grossest form led to the most recent outbreaks, during the Second World War. Troops were mostly protected by delousing, but the unfortunate victims of the concentration camps were not so lucky.

9 **Typhoid,** caused by *Salmonella typhimurium,* is, like cholera, spread by contaminated water and food. Engineers like Bazalgette vanquished this disease in the West by separating sewage and water supplies; vaccination further reduced the burden during the wars

of the early 20th century. The introduction of clean, filtered, chlorinated water into American cities in the late 19th and early 20th centuries led to a 90 per cent reduction in mortality, from 100 per 100,000 in 1890 to 7 per 100,000 by 1918. The name Mary Mallon will forever be associated with typhoid; this was the 'Typhoid Mary' who, as a symptomless carrier of the disease in 1906, infected 33 and killed three in New York. By 1936 the disease was virtually eradicated from the United States. There is an uncomfortable comparison with the developing world – in Pakistan in 1997 it was still the fourth commonest cause of death after perinatal deaths, heart attacks and diarrhoea.

10 **Tuberculosis** is now considered a global emergency by the WHO, killing between 2 and 3 million per year. One-third of the world's population is said to be infected. This is the epidemic that seemed to have a peculiar predilection for the famous and poetic; it has even acquired an unwarranted reputation for being a 'romantic' disease.

I should like to include two further epidemics on my list, one because it is so new and different, the other because it is the new scourge of the West and is undeniably closely related to infectious diseases. The first is **allergies** and the phenomenon of auto-immunity; as we shall see, cancers are closely related to this category. Finally, although the number of people actually killed by the epidemic of the **prion diseases BSE/vCJD** has to date been relatively small, this is the newest of our agents and is quite different from every other infectious disease. It also had catastrophic economic consequences for traditional farming communities in Britain and Europe.

We shall now proceed to examine types of epidemic, considering them by the nature of the agents that cause them. We shall commence with the life-form that is causing us most anxiety at the present, the virus.

CHAPTER 1

VIRUSES

Old sock, new sock

There is a conundrum taught to students of philosophy concerning socks. It is believed to have originated with John Locke (1632–1704). He asked us to imagine a new sock, and then imagine a sock that had been repaired by darning with fresh thread. Eventually every part of the sock wears out and is replaced with new thread. Locke's question is: what is the eventual product? Is it his original sock? Or a completely new one? Another version of the same puzzle involves an axe whose head and shaft serially need replacing. The same could be said to apply to humans and viruses, as we shall see.

Jenny was 23 and attended a Genito-Urinary Medicine clinic, very embarrassed, with severe pain and blistering around her genitals. Making a diagnosis of herpes was straightforward enough. This is a common sexually transmitted infection; we confirmed it with a simple swab sent to the virology lab, which subjected it to DNA tests. Treatment is simple enough too; there is a very safe and effective drug called acyclovir which stops the virus from reproducing. Poor Jenny proceeded to develop an unpleasant complication a day or so later; she abruptly stopped being able to pee properly, and had to come into hospital for a temporary catheter to be inserted in her bladder.

Herpes has achieved epidemic proportions in the West: it is five times as common as it was 20 years ago and affects 45 million Americans. Jenny will have a further long-term worry about this infection; she will never lose it. It will lie dormant in her nerve tissues and may reactivate intermittently for the rest of her life. The virus is immortalised in her nervous tissue, whether or not it reactivates. To an extent Jenny is now made of the herpes virus, like the very first new thread of Locke's sock.

There is a fine variety of traditional woollen clothing hand-made in Ireland called an Aran sweater. It is a kind of pullover, with a very special difference. Into the pattern of the wool is knitted a series of patterns – ropes, chains, diamonds and even more complicated knot designs. The function of the sweater was only partly the usual combination of weather protection and aesthetics. The people of Aran and neighbouring islands of the harsh northern Atlantic historically earned their living from the cruel sea; they were fishermen, mostly. Inevitably now and again there would be accidental drownings. In severe weather it might be some months or longer before a corpse was washed up. By then the features of the face might be unrecognisable, after long immersion in salt water. The wool sweater would most likely survive, and with it the knitted patterns carefully crafted in croft and cottage. Some say that by the exact pattern of cable and chain the poor drowned victim could be identified. It is also said that the craft is more exact still; family histories were recorded in wool in an easily decipherable, visible form.

This traditional skill, driven by hard necessity, precisely resembles the construction of the human genome. Examination of the individual fibres of wool reveals almost nothing. Similarly, determining the exact sequence of bases in the DNA spiral gives almost no information, beyond the nature of the substances that compose it. However, taking a step back and examining the patterns reveals the richness woven into them. Here is the history of the wearer, his ancestry recorded in otherwise inert material. Much of the intricacy of the pattern is redundant. Simple initials and date of birth would probably be adequate to identify most fishermen. However, a craft has evolved where redundancy is part and parcel of the final product, simultaneously pointless and vital. Now the vast majority of Aran sweaters are made without anyone really remembering their historical origins; certainly very few corpses of fishermen are now identified by the precise patterns of knitting in their sweaters.

So it is with genes. Initially the astounding discovery by Watson, Crick and their colleagues that our very being is constructed of inert bases was held to be the key to life. As science advances, so our previous understanding of how we arose shifts. Exactly like the Aran sweater, the design of any genome reflects the demands of the world in which the organism exists. It also contains huge amounts of redundancy, of apparent irrelevance, as though the designer of the blueprint had intermittently forgotten why she was doing it.

The Human Genome Project identified every shared sequence of bases in the DNA code that is common to all humans. A consequence of this project, which was made possible only because of the massive processing power of modern computers, was the characterisation of patterns of gene. Superficially, the DNA code is an apparently random series of four chemicals, or bases, stretching for almost unimaginable lengths along a double helical frame and arranged into chromosomes. However, the code is, of course, very far from random. Single mutations at crucial sites can have catastrophic consequences. There is, though, plenty of redundancy within DNA – a very high proportion of our genome is never expressed. Within those apparently useless segments there is some fascinating information to be mined. Some of the discoveries we have made have been absolutely startling.

The chimp and you

Pattern recognition of recognisable sequences has permitted us to compare our genes with those of other life forms with which we share our planet. Some are so similar to existing genetic material as to be indistinguishable, and with a consistency and regularity that simply could not have arisen by chance. The Animal Rights movement have already lit on this, and the phrase 'Chimpanzees share 95% of our genes' appears on many T-shirts (to which my response is – well, the other 5 per cent must be very important, to make us so different from chimpanzees). But we share genetic material with other life forms, and in a far stranger way. We have discovered to our surprise that up to 45 per cent of our genes are derived from what we might call 'mobile genetic elements'.

DNA is readily shuttled between organisms in bacteria. We have known this for many years. Indeed, we are facing the consequences of the promiscuity of genetic information between bacteria in the form of antibiotic resistance. Bacteria are readily capable of transferring genes that encode the processes that inactivate drugs. They do so not simply within the same species, but across species. Thus *Klebsiella* can acquire the genes for resistance to an antibiotic like gentamicin from an entirely different species such as *E. Coli*. One of the methods it uses is called the plasmid. This is simply a packet of DNA contained in a protein coat, which can be absorbed and incorporated by another bacterium. There are many further variants, some of which have splicing capacity for inserting their gene sequences in precisely the right place in the recipient's genome. Integrons, pathogenicity islands, transposons, retrotransposons and plasmids are all examples, each with a slightly different design and function.

The function of our nuclei (and equivalent structures in organisms like bacteria that do not have nuclei) is the efficient reproduction of DNA. To an extent, the mechanism by which this occurs is 'blind'. If presented with a recognisable sequence of DNA, the relevant enzymes – DNA polymerases – will reproduce it, and in humans they do so with astonishing fidelity. Thus we are sitting ducks for acquiring new genes through mobile genetic elements. As I have said, pattern recognition has demonstrated that a whopping 45 per cent of our genes are composed of such material. In other words entire segments of DNA have been incorporated into our chromosomes by whole-sale insertion, rather than by the slower process of selective evolution that we once believed determined our heredity.

What is Jenny now made of? Nearly half of her genes are 'mobile genetic elements'. Now, a little more of her is made of virus, in the form of herpes immortalised in her nervous tissue. Almost certainly she will have encountered other viruses, and will have genes from those episodes perpetually stored in her DNA. There is, actually, a difference between the mobile genetic elements and the genes she has acquired through infec-tions during her life; her children will not inherit the herpes genes (unless she infects them during birth, as sometimes happens); even then these herpes genes will not be passed on to her grandchildren.

This is an astonishing recent discovery. It has long been known that some infections may be passed from mother to child. HIV, hepatitis B, herpes, gonorrhoea and syphilis are part of a long list of such infections. The method of transmission here is quite different. These mobile genetic elements have become immor-talised in the parents, such that they are passed down the generations; the crucial difference is that the 'germ' cells – eggs and sperm – contain the material. Still, rather like Locke's sock it is hard to say where Jenny begins and the viruses and bacteria end. Jenny is made of an epidemic; in fact she is made of a series of epidemics.

There is more. Some of these genetic sequences resemble more than just mobile genetic elements: they were clearly once viruses. Scientists are now realising that many human genes are actually viral DNA. A recent estimate is that perhaps 50,000 or more viral sequences have entered the human genome. Many of these are retroviruses, much like the HIV/AIDS agent. At present most of these are believed to be 'silent' or inactive. We shall return to these, and to their effects, as some are involved in both health and disease. Much of this information has been derived from our understanding of the structure of the HIV. To the already startling fact that 45 per cent of our genes are derived from non-human mobile genetic elements we may now add that 8 per cent of our genes are composed of retroviruses almost identical to HIV. We know this because we can hunt out the gene patterns that result in, say, the viral envelope protein or other viral enzymes. These are the human endogenous retroviruses, or HERVs. Jenny's children will inherit HERVs and other mobile genetic elements present in both parents.

Thus we *are* viral material. Many questions arise about the presence of these viruses in our very being. Why have they been permitted to persist if they serve no function? One answer may be that eliminating them requires more energy expenditure than allowing them to persist. Another is that they do, in fact, have some use. There is increasing evidence that HERVs are not completely inert. Some whole proteins encoded by HERV genes are used for our benefit; there is a protein called syncytin, which helps cells stick together, which is unquestionably of HERV origin. There are others – interestingly, some vital for the attachment of the placenta to the womb, and thus vital to our survival as a species – and as our understanding progresses, more will be found.

Not all of the consequences of HERV infection are benign, though. Patterns of HERVs do seem to be associated with particular diseases. It is becoming increasingly clear that some groups of HERVs are more common with some cancers. Indeed, one of the first HERVs to be identified was initially known as the mouse mammary tumour virus. Other patterns may be associated with auto-immune diseases, and some even with psychiatric illnesses such as schizophrenia. The methods by which they act are considered in the chapter on auto-immune diseases and cancer. There has been an evolutionary trade-off between the relative benefits of accumulating viral material, with potentially useful genes attached, and these possibly dangerous consequences of infection.

The existence of HERVs and other microbially derived genes in our chromosomes gives rise to some striking speculation about the nature of our being. On the one hand we are a reflection of the environment in which we evolved. Our genes have evolved as a consequence of multiple challenges, including infections. On the other, we are actually partly composed of exactly that infectious material. How did these HERVs get into our genes? To answer that question, and to address the deeper issue central to this book, which is that we are composed of infectious material, we must ask, what is a virus?

What a virus is

The straightforward scientific answer is that a virus is a packet of infectious genetic material. As such it is almost – but not quite – the odd one out in our list of agents of epidemics, in that it lacks an important property. Bacteria, fungi and parasites are at least in part capable of independent reproduction. I exclude from this definition those parasites that are dependent on specific hosts to ensure their reproduction. The human malaria parasite, for instance, cannot reproduce without both mosquitoes and humans. Nevertheless it contains the machinery necessary for the task within its own structures. This is quite different from the nature of viruses. There are also some bacteria that behave in a similar way to viruses, requiring some constituents of the host to survive and reproduce. The existence of 'half-way houses' does not challenge the definition. It simply illustrates the capacity of different types of organisms to explore evolutionary niches. The other exception is the Creutzfeldt-Jakob disease agent, the prion (previously known as a slow virus), and we shall discuss that in Chapter 8.

Viruses can survive but not reproduce on inanimate objects. Research in cancer and haematology wards has demonstrated viable virus on all kinds of materials, including doors and handles, but the virus cannot multiply in that state. This capacity to survive on non-living material is very important in the transmission of epidemics like SARS and influenza, but viruses can only truly exist by hijacking the machinery of some other living organism in order to reproduce. That living organism may be the most primitive single-celled amoeba, or may be a plant or a higher animal, but without such a host the virus is at a dead end.

The simplest viruses are short sequences of genetic material contained in a protein envelope, which is itself made by the victim, as it is forced to do by the virus' genes. That envelope will have some means of attaching to the cells of its host and of entering the cell. In essence that is all a virus comprises and requires. Some viruses – HIV, for instance – may contain some of the machinery required for their own reproduction in the form of enzymes, but the point remains valid. The virus cannot reproduce unless it is inside a host cell.

That essential feature of their nature poses a further philosophical question about them. Are they actually alive? Anyone who has had a viral infection (which means everyone) will be in little doubt that they were at the mercy of a living thing, particularly if they passed it on to someone else. However, it is only very recently in our history that such a hypothesis has been confirmed. Viruses are so reliant upon other organisms for their survival that their definition is almost oxymoronic. A virus is something that is only truly active when it infects something else. That infection may or may not result in disease – and as we have seen it may be beneficial – but the definition of a virus is only truly complete in the context of its infected host.

What definition would satisfy an independent observer that any particle of tissue was alive? One is the consumption of nutrients and the emission of waste products. Such a definition is routinely invoked by scientists searching for evidence of life on other planets. Trace quantities of organic waste products such as methane or carbon dioxide would be taken, if not as proof, as convincing corroborative evidence that life was or had been present. Viruses do not either consume nutrients or emit waste. All of their synthetic processes, all of their energy requirements, are provided by the host cell. Any waste products are similarly produced by the same cells, not by the virus itself. Those waste products may be different from 'normal' because of the viral infection, but it is still not the virus that is emitting them. A planet populated entirely by viruses would therefore appear entirely lifeless to NASA. Of course, by our definition above, such a state of affairs could not arise. The virus would need hosts, and our NASA scientists would detect the waste products of our virus' hosts.

Oddly enough, the definition of a virus is very close to properties we rely on for our own survival. It would be a brave scientist who claimed that sperm were not living things. Yet a spermatozoon, although it passes the test of consuming nutrients and emitting waste products, is not of course complete in the sense of being able to reproduce itself, until it 'infects' an egg. In this respect sperm are closer to viruses, although because they contain the machinery required for their own metabolism they are otherwise closer to bacteria. Sperm have to attach and fuse to the egg in order to fertilise it. The process by which they do so is almost identical, and uses the same protein types, as the process used by viruses fusing with the cells of their victims.

There is more. Sperm have a major and significant difference from both viruses and bacteria. They have a separate, walled-off nucleus in which their delicate DNA is protected. The reason sperm have this nucleus is at least in part to protect it from the dangerous properties of an ancient infectious, bacterial invader which all higher organisms share. We shall return to this in our chapter on bacteria; for the moment I shall simply name the invader. It is called the mitochondrion. I mention it here because the female ovum treats the invading sperm mitochondria exactly as any other cell would an infecting bacterium – it kills them. As a consequence all human mitochondria are derived from the female line, and we can see that the moment of conception is very similar to an 'infection'.

Life on our planet is susceptible to infectious epidemics because life itself evolved through infection. For humans and higher animals that reproduce through sex, that includes the 'infection' of the unfertilised ovum by sperm. As is now clear, that 'infection' begins before we are born, at conception. It actually began even earlier, before humans and higher animals appeared on the planet. At an even deeper level we are all made of the same stuff as infectious diseases. Taken at its most basic, this simply means that our essential blueprint is shared. All life forms – except prions – have the same chemical building blocks, the nucleic acids. These are arranged as chains of either DNA or RNA. As we shall repeatedly see, the properties we share are far more closely allied than even this.

What viruses do

In the context of viruses, once these chains of DNA or RNA are released into the cell they can behave in a number of ways. They may do nothing at all. They may kill the cell, having forced its machinery to make copies of itself. They may remain in the cell but redirect that same machinery to their own reproductive ends without killing it. In the case of some common viral diseases – chicken pox, measles – the virus may reactivate months or even decades later. Some viruses may so disrupt the reproductive machinery of the cell that they cause cancer. However, some may also become latent and incorporate permanently into the genes of the host. In the case of some viruses this incorporation may be harmless, or even beneficial, and as we have said, it can be passed from mother to offspring. These properties of viruses explain much of their capacity to cause epidemics. Their similarity to us, and the fact that we are partly composed of material indistinguishable from viruses, makes us sitting ducks for viral assault.

The freedom from the need to fuel and monitor their own reproduction allows viruses one much more crucial property. It permits a much greater capacity for mutation. Higher organisms that reproduce for themselves need to ensure faithful copying of their blueprint into the next generation. Defective cells will not function properly, and the animal may die as a consequence. They – we – therefore rely on a 'proof-reading' mechanism. The chances of a mutational error creeping in when your and my cells reproduce is lower than the order of one in a billion. Viruses are far sloppier. So long as they can enter a cell and reproduce they are 'happy'. A single virus may produce many thousands of offspring in a single cell. If a few mutations creep in, so what?

Finding ancestors

Where do viruses come from? In the evolutionary sense this is a very difficult question to answer. We cannot look to a fossil record to examine their origins. They are too fragile and small to persist in fossilised tissue, and to date no virus has ever been identified in this state. We have already seen that viruses cannot really exist except in the context of their hosts. It therefore seems reasonable that we can place the chicken of life before the egg of viruses; however, this may be completely wrong, as we shall see later.

We can take another approach. We can examine the huge number of viruses that have been identified and compare their structure. This allows us to plot evolutionary trees and attempt to speculate about a common ancestor. This even allows us some information about the date at which particular viruses might have emerged. I shall illustrate this by an analogy. Suppose you live in a Victorian house and you wish to know exactly when it was built, but the deeds have been lost. You might notice that details of the structure of your house are slightly different from those of some houses in the neighbouring area, but similar or identical to those of others. Victorian developments tended to be built street-by-street, and the builders might have bought job lots of stained glass for the front door or tiling for the hallway. If you compare your house with others that show the same features, the architectural details will allow you to make a very accurate estimate of the date of construction.

Exactly the same technique may be used with viruses. This has been possible since even before modern technology allowed us to sequence entire genes. It has long been known that groups of viruses vary far more than higher organisms in their blueprints. Unlike more advanced life-forms, some viruses have genes made of RNA rather than DNA. The arrangement of the genes varies hugely between viral types, as does the structure of the protein envelope. All of this information, when combined, compared and collated, has allowed us to make a speculation about the precise origin of the first ever virus.

The conclusion that has been drawn is that there wasn't one. We are a little limited in our complete analysis because by far the bulk of our knowledge derives from viruses that infect land-based life-forms. That is a serious limitation. Viruses infect every known true life-form. Seawater is teeming with viruses to such a degree that growth of plankton is considered to be restricted by them. If we compare our comparative ignorance of the huge number and variety of viruses that occur in seawater with our knowledge of bacteria, the scale of the missing data is revealed. Only about 10 per cent of the bacteria we recover from seawater belong to any recognised existing grouping. Extrapolate that to the vast range of non-bacterial organisms that inhabit the oceans, all of which will almost certainly harbour viruses, and you will appreciate the scale of the problem.

Nevertheless the huge diversity in the structure of viruses we have already identified suggests that they probably did not share a single common ancestor. This is not surprising when we return to our definition of a virus. These infections co-evolved with their hosts, by necessity. They cannot reproduce without them, and therefore each will adapt to the type of organism it infects. The diversity of viruses reflects the diversity of life on the planet. When life emerged from the sea in the form of bacteria 3,500 million years ago, the emerging life-forms brought viruses with them. As evolution progressed, viruses persisted – and adapted – keeping pace with the huge number of new opportunities that presented themselves.

Bottoms and tops

There are conflicting theories about the nature of viruses before they assumed the incomplete, reproductively incapable forms I am describing. One we might call the bottom-up theory, the other the top-down. The top-down theory maintains that viruses are stripped-down parasites. At one time in their evolutionary history they were more complete organisms, with all the necessary equipment to generate their own energy and reproduce. Some of these parasites found that they could survive in a simpler form and shed their redundant, metabolically expensive apparatus.

It is of note here that bacteria are capable of emitting those small protein-bound packets of DNA we encountered above called mobile genetic elements, of which there are a number of types including plasmids. They can be absorbed by other bacteria, usually but not always of the same species. Such structures are extremely important in our war against bacteria, as we shall discover, and to our own essence. In some respects these plasmids, being a sequence of genetic material in an envelope, are identical to viruses. It is entirely possible that something resembling a plasmid was the first-ever virus. A plasmid encoding only genes that govern its own reproduction might have stumbled into a new host and hijacked its machinery. It was then able to reproduce the process and itself.

The contrasting bottom-up theory refers to the ability of organic chemicals to spontaneously order themselves. Put simply, this means that inert compounds have the capacity to arrange themselves in a manner very similar to the basic building blocks of life. Scientists such as Miller, Urey and Juan Oro performed astonishing – if controversial – experiments in the 1950s and 1960s which hinted at the very origins of life itself. They attempted to reproduce what they believed were the chemicals present in the earth's atmosphere prior to the emergence of life, and then subjected them to electrical energy. Such energy would have been present in pre-life earth in the form of thunderstorms and lightning. They discovered that a remarkable array of organic compounds resulted. Oro was even able to produce the vital base adenine by a similar experiment. In 1957 Heinz Fraenkel-Conrat and R C Williams demonstrated that viruses can 'self-assemble' in exactly the same way. They broke up a virus into its two parts, the RNA and the envelope. When they put the parts back together again, they reformed into active virus. *Viruses can self-assemble, exactly like the organic compounds of the Miller-Urey experiment.*

You may be thinking at this moment, so what? What difference does this make in a book about epidemics? Here's what. Adenine is one of the key 'bases' that make up both DNA and RNA. Amino acids are the building blocks of proteins, and are also capable of self-assembly. In other words, the majority of the essential components of a virus can spontaneously self-assemble in the right environmental conditions. The same building-blocks are also the basis of all known life-forms except prions. If this theory is correct, then 'life' and something indistinguishable from a virus – a packet of DNA or RNA in a protein coat – arose at the same time and from the same ancestor. Here is another sense in which *we are viruses, because we may have evolved from them.* Once again, it is not surprising that we become victims of something almost indistinguishable from our own essence.

The virus from outer space

I should now deal briefly with a further hypothesis, which suggests that viruses may have arrived on our planet on the vehicle of a meteorite or other matter from outer space. Such theories were widespread at the time when the AIDS pandemic emerged. A major objection to them is that viruses are susceptible to radiation, ultra-violet light and heat. Space is rich in radiation and ultra-violet light, and entry into our atmosphere is a potent source of heat, so it is unlikely that viruses could have survived this journey. A further source of doubt concerns the nature of viruses. Who were their hosts before they hitched their ride? It is theoretically possible that a virus (or similar, related structure) could survive deep within a meteorite, but its survival would rely on thousands of years of dormancy after leaving its original planet.

Some meteorites have, though, been shown to be rich in the sorts of amino acids that Juan Oro was able to generate in his pre-life experiment. A meteorite that landed in Murchison, Australia in 1969 contained over 90 different amino acids. Nineteen of these amino acids are found on Earth. The earth's crust is pocked with the evidence of such collisions, and they are often much larger. It is thus possible that the fabric of 'life'– and therefore viruses – arrived with a meteorite. The significance of this is that once again the conclusion would be drawn that we all share a common ancestor. We are viruses; we are epidemics.

The species jumper

Whichever of the theories you choose to believe, it is undeniably the case that all species co-evolved with viruses, and that generally viruses are restricted to a single species. That is not the full story, though, and to understand human epidemics with viruses we need to understand a further layer of complexity in the analysis of viral evolution. Viruses can and do jump species barriers. This is of crucial importance in our understanding of the nature and origins of epidemics of viral infections, particularly the 'newer' ones such as West Nile fever, HIV, and the episodes of avian influenza which have arisen in humans so far.

At first sight the fact that viruses can leap from one species to another may seem to contradict one of the key characteristics of a virus. For infection to occur, the outer envelope of the virus has to bind to a receptor on the cell of its victim. These receptors are generally specific, like a lock and its key. Jenny's herpes virus, for instance, can only infect humans, and its receptor binds almost exclusively to nerve tissue, which explains why it tends to recur only in specific sites. The HIV agent only binds to certain kinds of immune cells, and all of its effects may be predicted from the fact that it is so restricted. Thus animal and plant viruses generally tend to be restricted to their particular animal and plant host. This would seem to be an inevitable consequence of the route the viruses have taken in their evolution. As host and invader co-evolved they have become intimately and inextricably co-dependent. However, viruses can indeed jump from species to species. For this to occur another property of viruses must be invoked. That property is their capacity for mutation.

Certain types of virus are more efficient in this respect than others. Hepatitis C, a virus that is causing a worldwide epidemic of liver infection, is presently believed to be entirely restricted to humans. HIV, although apparently restricted to humans, has a phenomenal capacity for mutation, such that no two viruses are ever identical, even if taken from the same human. Influenza A is peculiarly capable of mutation for reasons related to its structure, and infects many different animal species. We shall discuss this in more detail in the relevant section, but one of the primary reasons that we are so concerned about the possibility of a global pandemic of influenza A is, in part, this skill in mutation.

Mutation is not absolutely and always a necessity. The ability of viruses to cross the species barrier is also related to the intensity of exposure. So far the deaths from avian influenza among humans have almost exclusively been among people who have handled infected birds or animals. Sufficiently intimate and sustained contact with the virus seems to permit invasion despite an imperfect match between the viral protein and its host receptor. Nor is this the only example. The current leading theory about how HIV came to infect humans is based on this principle. A similar virus infects apes, particularly chimpanzees. It is now believed that apes butchered for bushmeat were infected with simian immunodeficiency virus (SIV), which bypassed some of the natural defence mechanisms of human skin in tiny abrasions caused during the bloody mechanical process.

A virus that successfully invades a new species host can take a number of paths. It might cause no illness. It might make the host ill, but in an evolutionary sense be at a dead end, because it still cannot readily transmit to another host of the same species. However, it can also adapt within the new species. There are two methods by which it may do so. In the case of HIV it is believed – but by no means certain – that the virus spontaneously mutated to survive and transmit between humans.

Other viruses take advantage of a different method, co-infection. Two influenza viruses present in the same animal can swap genes. This is one source of anxiety in the context of influenza. Imagine, for example, a duck strain and a pig strain being present in the same animal. Shuffling of genes can then occur between the two viral strains. The consequence is a third, hybrid virus which may have a much wider capacity to infect numerous different species – including humans.

A virus may also infect a new species by hitching a ride with a biting insect or tick. Rather like our example of SIV first infecting humans after having broken through the barrier of the skin, an insect can inject viral particles directly into the bloodstream. Much is made of the remarkable adaptability of our immune system, with its complexity of white blood cell types and immune proteins that identify and neutralise infection. In fact for real protection from infectious disease our primary defences are far more important. These are simple mechanisms such as our tough skin, oily secretions, nostril hairs, tears and sweat that keep would-be invaders at bay. These are like the walls of our castle. Once breached, the garrison might or might not be able to annihilate the enemy. It's far better, though, never to let them in at all.

Our so-called 'innate' immune system comprises our castle's walls. In fact it is more complex and sophisticated than simply mechanical obstruction, but once an invader is past it, it becomes useless. There are many viruses that take this route. Yellow fever is an excellent example. Indeed, many of the newer diseases such as Nipah and Hendra which have recently troubled us are carried by biting insects. It is not hard to see why. As humans encroach ever deeper into animal habitats and disrupt the local ecology, both insects and viruses encounter new hosts. We shall encounter this rather worrying phenomenon later.

If this were a textbook of infectious diseases and epidemiology, I would proceed at this point to subdivide viral types and discuss the illnesses they cause. I do not intend to take this route, because I believe that the differences between, say, a flavivirus and a picornavirus are of little interest to the general reader. I shall, however, discuss a few key moments in the history of the discovery of viruses.

Learning the enemy

The first depiction of any kind of a virus was, predictably, concerned with its effect rather than the agent itself. The science of virology arose later than its cousin bacteriology, simply because most viruses evaded the scrutiny of the primitive light microscopes which began to appear in the 17th century. That did not prevent the ancient Egyptians from illustrating the effects of viral infection in a hieroglyph dated 3700 BC. The image is of the priest Ruma, and clearly shows the withered leg of a sufferer from polio. A mummy excavated in 1905 containing the body of the Pharaoh Siptah, dating from the 12th century BC, showed unequivocal evidence of the same disease. The body of Rameses V when unwrapped showed clear evidence of smallpox, almost certainly the cause of his death in 1143 BC.

The first intervention between man and viral disease arose almost 3,000 years before anything even faintly resembling a virus was identified. There is clear documentary evidence that the Chinese have practised variolation – inoculation of matter, or pus, from the active pock-marks of sufferers from mild smallpox – since about 1000 BC. Mild smallpox is also known by its Brazilian name of alastrim. There are three points of note about this practice. The first is that it continued intermittently for almost 3,000 years until true vaccination was discovered in south-west England in the 18th century. Indeed, supporters of variolation were implacably opposed to Edward Jenner's revolutionary 18th century smallpox vaccine. The second is the principle, vital to our understanding of epidemics and how we might control them, that even fatal diseases like smallpox can vary in their severity. The final point is that exposure to a modified or less virulent strain of a virus or a related strain confers lasting immunity to that virus. It is a rich quirk of history that the first two viral illnesses to show their faces in enduring human records – smallpox and polio – are also the two that humankind has had the best chance of eradicating through such vaccination.

The notion that identifiable 'germs' cause disease is an astonishingly recent development in our collective history. Although many ancient civilisations practised quarantine, and had sewer drainage, public lavatories and fresh water supplies, they had no better understanding of what actually caused illness than they had of the composition of the moon. The most widely held belief was that illness was a divine visitation for conscious or unconscious sin. Sometimes contaminated air was blamed. The word 'malaria' derives from the Spanish for 'bad air', a far guess from the reality of mosquitoes and *Plasmodium* parasites. It was not until the 19th century that Robert Koch and Louis Pasteur developed the theory that we now accept without qualm – that infections are caused by tiny life-forms.

Even though by 1885 Pasteur had developed a vaccine for rabies, and hepatitis had been shown to be infectious, the concept of a virus was still unknown. A clue came the following year. A British pathologist called John Buist noticed what he called 'elementary bodies' while examining lymph tissue from a smallpox victim under a microscope. He believed he had identified tiny bacteria. We now know that these were pox virus particles. The viruses of the pox group – of which there are a number, one of which, cowpox, has proven vital to our modern health – are easily the largest of those that afflict humankind. They are just visible under the light microscope.

Virology did not properly emerge as a science until 1892, and even then the significance of the discovery was not properly realised, partly because the findings were believed to apply only within botany. A Russian scientist called Iwanowski demonstrated that a disease of tobacco plants could be transmitted from infected to uninfected leaves despite filtration through ceramic filters too fine to permit passage of the smallest known bacteria. The baton was taken up in 1898 by a brilliant Dutch soil microbiologist called Professor M W Beijerinck. He called the infectious agent *contagium vivum fluidum* ('soluble living germ'). In the same year it was realised that foot-and-mouth disease in cattle was caused by a similar filterable agent. However, the scientific community at large still rejected the hypothesis that these invisible and occult entities could be the cause of disease in humans.

It was only at the very threshold of the 20th century that the doctrine of a 'virus' causing illness began to gain acceptance. Yet the word 'virus' is an ancient one. In Latin it meant 'a slimy liquid, poison, offensive odour or taste'. The word appears in Lanfranc's *Cirurgie*, written about 1400, in its exact Latin sense. It began to appear in medical journals during the 18th century, but in the sense of any noxious fluid. Cleopatra was held to have succumbed to the 'virus of an asp' in Mead's *Poisons* of 1702. With what must be accidental but uncanny prophecy, there is a quotation from the *British Medical Journal* of 1800 which reads: 'the pustules … contain a perfect Small-pox virus'. This was almost 100 years before Buist observed his elemental bodies.

Only from about 1900 onwards, when Walter Reed of the US Military demonstrated the route of transmission of yellow fever, did the word begin to assume a more specific definition, close to the one we examined above. Coincidentally, in the *Journal of the American Medical Association* of 1900 there was an article published by an Italian team categorically refuting that yellow fever is caused by a virus. It was to be a further 37 years before the virus could be grown – in chick embryos, by Max Theiler, who also developed the vaccine which is still in use.

The first disease to be conclusively demonstrated to be caused by a virus in humans and animals was polio. Karl Landsteiner ground up the spinal tissue of children who had died of the disease and used it to transmit the disease to apes. Yet viruses were not properly visualised, even indirectly, until 1935, when Wendell Stanley crystallised Tobacco Mosaic Virus (TMV) and showed that it remains infectious – a discovery which earned him the Nobel Prize. In 1940 viruses were properly observed for the first time when Helmuth Ruska managed to image them using an electron microscope.

Catching up with bacteriology

I have dwelt on the early development of virology as a science for a number of reasons. The first is to demonstrate how recently viruses have revealed their nature to us. It is often said that virology is 50 years behind bacteriology, although that gap is rapidly closing. Since Iwanowski's seminal if initially neglected observations the science of virology has accelerated apace, although it is still not quite as advanced as bacteriology in at least one significant respect. Unlike bacterial diseases, there are a significant number of viral illnesses for which there is as yet no effective treatment. While a small number of bacteria have become untreatable, for a variety of reasons, by and large there are successful antibiotics for just about all of them. The story with respect to viruses is not so straightforward.

Yellow fever, Lassa, Marburg, Ebola, human T-cell lymphotropic virus, measles, human papilloma virus, hepatitis A, B, C, D and E, rubella, mumps, polio, Epstein Barr Virus and many more – none has a completely reliable and targeted treatment. Many are preventable through vaccination, but once the diseases they cause are established there are only limited options that the medical profession has to offer. The reason for this relates to our initial definition of the nature and function of viruses. To reproduce, a virus has to incorporate into the cell and even the genes of its host – it has to become part of us, like Locke's sock. It is clearly a major challenge to destroy an invader which has become so intimately integrated into the essence of its victim, without the possibility of serious 'friendly fire' damaging innocent tissue.

The second point about viruses and science is that some of our most successful interventions were developed long before the nature of viruses was fully understood. The most successful vaccine of all time – for smallpox – was developed about 100 years before Buist first even glimpsed the organism. To an extent, the science we have developed may even hinder us in controlling viral epidemics. We should nervously note a salient feature of the WHO's foremost success in eradicating smallpox – that we could not repeat that success today, at least not by the same means. The methods that Jenner used were far too bold and radical for our risk-averse age (see pages 72–75).

The same rule applies to other giant strides made in virology. Pasteur saved lives with his rabies vaccine 50 years before the first virus was even visualised, using methods that would nowadays be considered impossibly hazardous. Reed and Agremont demonstrated the route of transmission of yellow fever in experiments that would probably result in criminal proceedings in the modern world; they deliberately inoculated a passing soldier with yellow fever using a captive mosquito. The control of modern epidemics – viral or otherwise – is based on public health and containment principles that were established in the 19th century. Put simply, we knew how to deal with many viruses before we even knew what a virus was, and we rely on the findings of a bolder, less risk-averse age.

The newer science of virology has nevertheless yielded some impressive therapies. The most notable in this regard is the very recent development of combination therapy for HIV. This has revolutionised our management of this most recent and disastrous of epidemics. The drugs that have been developed have relied on sophisticated understanding of precise mechanisms of viral activity. This would not have been possible in Pasteur's time, nor would he have been able to develop a vaccine by the methods he used for rabies. Indeed, a vaccine for HIV continues to elude us despite our ability to examine the agent of this extraordinary and catastrophic scourge in the minutest of detail.

The big one

Now we have discussed the nature of viruses, and illustrated how new the science of virology is, it is time to address individually the viruses that we fear for their epidemic potential. Later in this book we shall discuss how some diseases have become more 'fashionable' than others, and therefore attract more research funding and public attention. Rather in that vein, I shall begin by discussing what is currently the most topical of the viral epidemics – influenza.

Rather like a bioterrorist's threat, influenza has had the remarkable effect of causing worldwide public anxiety without as yet causing mass casualties. Much of the source of this international stress lies within the scientific community. Generally scientists try to avoid sensationalism and mass panic. How is it that – at the time of writing – they have so agitated us that the nests of migratory birds and swans in public parks are being attacked by terrified humans?

The statistic that the global influenza pandemic of 1918–20 killed more people than the First World War surely explains much of the concerns of experts. There were other pandemics in the 20th century, although none of the scale of this so-called Spanish flu. In 1957 and 1958 the Asian flu epidemic killed 'only' 69,800 in the United States alone. Between September 1968 and March 1969 the Hong Kong pandemic had a death toll of 33,800, making it the mildest pandemic of the 20th century. Were we to plot this on a graph we would readily see that a further outbreak is overdue; the most pessimistic prediction might be that we could see another pandemic with mass casualties on the scale of 1918–20.

History, though, is a necessary but insufficient source of anxiety about another influenza outbreak. All epidemics and pandemics tend to follow cycles with peaks and troughs. Plague, cholera, typhoid, tuberculosis and measles all demonstrate the same phenomenon. It reflects a basic fact about epidemics of infection within populations – that an infectious disease will achieve a state of balance with its hosts until either a sufficient number of new victims with ineffective immunity is born, or the infection alters its nature to become more or less dangerous, or the vector (see Glossary, but for example the malaria mosquito) is controlled, or any combination of these things occurs.

We can examine how this comes about. The first happens because we have, in addition to the 'innate' immune system mentioned above, a more sophisticated 'adaptive' immune system. The innate branch of the system is generally not specific to any particular type of infection. Intact skin is as effective a barrier to any type of infection. The adaptive branch is directed and particular to the precise invading microbe.

Adaptive immunity

There are essentially two methods by which animals may naturally acquire adaptive immunity to an infection. The first is called 'passive'. Some immunity may be passed from a mother to her offspring, either across the placenta prior to birth or in breast milk. This immunity takes the form of antibodies. Antibodies are proteins produced by white blood cells, and they are specific and precise for a particular invader. When circulating freely they are usually inert. However, when they bind to their target – a portion of the infecting agent – they trigger activity in other immune cells to destroy the invader.

Passive immunity wanes comparatively quickly, in a matter of months. However, modern humankind can harness this ability by injecting purified antibodies. The old vaccine for hepatitis A was based on this principle, and once again the immunity provided by this route was transient. It can readily be seen that the antibody from the mother relies on one vital principle. *She must have encountered the infection, even if in vaccine form, in order to have antibodies to pass on.*

This leads us to our next source of naturally acquired, active, adaptive immunity, which is to contract the disease and survive. It is important to understand that even highly infectious and lethal diseases generally do not kill every single member of a population. Those exposed to infection who do not die as a result will develop immunity. Even those who do die will have embarked on the process, but not sufficiently effectively or quickly to protect themselves.

The ultimate final pathway of the successful kind of immunity is the same antibody that is passed from mother to offspring. The difference in this context is that a set of white blood cells will now have 'learnt' to produce the antibodies for themselves. This means that if the infection is acquired again, these cells will be waiting for it. They will be able to produce the antibody trigger in sufficient quantities and at a sufficient rate to destroy the infection.

Flu fights back

You might predict from the above that influenza should therefore pose no threat to humankind. It circulates naturally anyway with consequent widespread immunity; generally it causes short-lived if unpleasant symptoms; it kills only the infirm and the elderly. I have mentioned above, though, that two features can change the balance of infection versus immunity in a population. The first is adaptive immunity. The second is that the virus itself may change.

Here then is the nub. Influenza can and does change. In fact it changes in at least two ways, one of which is more dangerous than the other, although both are capable of killing, and both are capable of causing epidemics.

Influenza viruses are made of RNA. This is important, because RNA is more labile and prone to mutation than DNA. There are three main influenza groups, designated A, B and C. It is A that concerns us most as humans, although B also causes illness, which tends to be mild. The more dangerous influenza A mutates at a constant, steady rate, driven by its sloppy proof-reading. Every so often enough cumulative small mutations produce a virus that is sufficiently different from a regional strain to circumvent existing adaptive immunity and cause a localised epidemic. These vary in severity and extent, but do not approach the mass pandemics that cause scientists so much anxiety. This is called antigenic drift.

There are two key features that should be noted. The first is that sufficient 'cross-over' immunity from the previous viral strain protects the majority from severe disease, so that only the very old, the very young and those with other coincidental chronic illnesses like diabetes or renal failure are at risk of death. The second is that no animal intermediary is required to produce this change in the virus. Nevertheless minor mutants may cause significant epidemics and mortality.

The second method by which influenza A might become markedly more dangerous, and the one that worries us more, is called antigenic shift. This occurs because of two peculiarities of influenza. The first is that the virus is not confined to humans, and can affect a variety of animals including pigs, horses and migratory fowl. Generally in their wild, unadulterated form the viruses are confined by their lock-and-key binding mechanism to their animals of origin. The other is the configuration of its genes. The majority of viruses contain DNA or RNA in complete strands: sometimes double, sometimes single. Influenza contains nine separate RNA strands. For reasons that will become clear, they are rather like a hand of tarot cards dealt by a fortune teller.

Two different strands of virus may infect the same animal. This is not unexpected where livestock are housed together, or pigs roam near water courses where there are migratory birds, or in markets where animals are displayed and sold live. This frequently happens in the Far East, and certainly did at the Bull Ring camp at Etaples in 1916. The two hands of tarot may then be shuffled. Precisely as in tarot (although in a slightly more scientifically valid way!), the exact configuration of the resulting hybrid of the two packs determines what happens next. The hybrid virus might still be confined to, say, pigs and horses. It might be a harmless variety, which still causes infection but does so trivially. If, however, it contains the Death card in the correct configuration, then the virus might proceed to infect humans.

The exchange of our tarot cards requires a further refinement. This is based on the principle that some animals are more like us than others. Transplant surgeons looking for animal tissue to graft into humans select one particular species for that reason. The animal that serves humans best, for both transplant purposes and influenza transmission, is the pig. As Winston Churchill said, cats look down at us, dogs look up to us, but a pig regards us as its absolute equal. It is easier for us to contract influenza A from the humble swine than from just about any other animal. The reason for this is that the particular lock-and-key mechanism that allows influenza to invade human tissues is remarkably similar to that of the pig; humans are more like pigs than most other animals. The actual 'locks' are called sialic acid residues. They are principally located on the lining of the airways.

There are several potential properties to be kept in mind about our new strain of influenza. First, it will be equally as prone as any other influenza virus to minor mutation through antigenic drift. Thus a strain that initially only affects fowl without killing them might mutate through drift to become lethal to, for example, ducks or swans. Next, if the virus acquires the lock-and-key mechanism to affect a new species it will behave like a totally new infection within that species. As we have said, diseases to which our immunity has never been exposed tend to have a far higher mortality. Finally, the inability to infect a species that does not share the correct lock-and-key receptor mechanism may be overcome where exposure to the virus is sufficiently intimate.

We should also consider here the naming of parts. The world is currently most concerned with the H5N1 strain of influenza A. The H stands for haemagglutinin, the N for neuraminidase. To pursue our tarot analogy, H is the Chariot card, N the Death card. By this is meant that H transports the virus into the cell by binding via the lock-and-key mechanism already mentioned. N does the damage. This is a simplification, but for the purposes of understanding epidemics it will suffice. The numbers type the strains of the virus to their subsets; thus influenza A/Texas/77/H3N2 describes a strain identified in Texas in 1977 with the haemagglutinin/neuraminidase configuration H3N2.

A change in the nature of an infection like influenza illustrates one of the most important features in understanding epidemics, and one that is worth repeating for emphasis. That is this: *an infectious disease that is introduced to a previously unexposed population will behave entirely differently from the same disease in a population in which it is endemic.* This principle has affected the fates of entire nations and continents, following the introduction of viruses like smallpox and measles.

Our new virus has a further property in the context of vaccine-preventable disease, namely that a vaccine directed against a strain that has reconfigured by antigenic shift will be useless. I shall introduce a troubling problem here. We are presently concerned about a strain of influenza that is lethal to birds. Vaccines for flu are mass-produced in embryonated (that is living) hens' eggs. Can you foresee a problem here?

Bad colds and terrible influenzas

Most of us believe we have had flu at some point. If you are reading this now, of course you survived, as do most people who contract influenza each year. The currently circulating avian influenza strain has a mortality among humans of around 60 per cent. How can we balance these apparently contradictory observations?

The symptoms of genuine influenza are severe but not specific. They include agonising headaches, muscle pains, fevers, cough and prostration. In order to fit our true definition, laboratory evidence must also be present to confirm the diagnosis. The first point to be made is therefore that the diagnosis of flu is often incorrectly made. It is often facetiously said that women get colds, and men get flu. The implication is that illness tolerance among men is so much lower that they behave as though they have severe flu even when they have a mild common cold. Those of us who have taken a day or so off work and rung in saying we had flu probably didn't have it.

Among those who genuinely are infected by the influenza virus, there may be a number of different outcomes. Let us first consider routine, endemic influenza, of the sort that causes outbreaks and epidemics either by antigenic drift or by spilling over into a new population. We make this distinction from a totally different strain that arises from antigenic shift, because the outcomes are radically different. For the most part, the healthy and comparatively young, if unvaccinated, will have an unpleasant but short-lived illness of very abrupt onset from which they will recover. The onset may be so sudden that victims may be able to describe the exact hour at which they fell ill. They may appear very unwell, with a flushed, toxic appearance. Severe pain may result simply from moving the eyes. In children, muscle pain may be most prominent in the calves. For the most part the worst symptoms resolve themselves after three days, although a second bout of fever is common, and a runny nose, nasal obstruction and cough may persist for some further days before a full recovery is made, which can take one or two weeks.

Recovery is not universal, however. Endemic influenza can and does kill young, healthy people. The most common cause of death is pneumonia. This may happen either because there is a particularly virulent infection of the lungs by the virus itself, or because there is invasion of the damaged tissues by unrelated bacteria – usually staphylococci. Nor are these the only complications. Inflammation of the heart may sometimes arise, and influenza is a cause of the deadly Reye's syndrome, which leads to fatal infiltration of the brain and liver with fat tissue in children. Fortunately all of these are rare. The situation is different among the elderly, those with damaged immunity, or those with heart disease or kidney disease. For these groups even workaday flu can be fatal.

Now let us consider our new strain which has arisen by antigenic shift. This is effectively a completely new challenge to human immunity. Death may arise from any of the complications mentioned above, and in fact is more likely because the virus might replicate faster than white blood cells can control it. However, further complications may arise. In our battle for immunity against the virus a sort of arms race may break out.

Immunity works in part by the production of chemicals that activate white blood cells. In fact these chemicals – cytokines – are responsible for many of the symptoms of even uncomplicated flu. They are produced for a reason – they 'prime' immune cells to become active. We make use of this property in treating other viral infections. Interferon is one such chemical. It is used in attempting to eradicate a number of viruses, notably hepatitis C. During treatment patients often complain of symptoms identical to flu. The trigger to produce these cytokines is the presence of influenza-generated proteins on human cells. Where the trigger cannot be switched off, a catastrophic state of affairs arises where more and more toxic cytokines are produced and the body begins to damage itself. This is known as a 'cytokine storm'. It has more than one cause – other infections may cause it, as may massive trauma and burns.

A moment's thought will reveal an explanation for the paradox of pandemic influenza. It works in the opposite way from the trend for older, sicker people to become victims of viruses. Young, healthy immune systems are far more efficient at pumping out cytokines in toxic quantities. Such was the case in the Spanish flu outbreak of 1918–20.

Our new, reassorted virus might have other properties that increase its lethality. Ordinary epidemic flu binds to our lock-and-key receptors in the respiratory tract and generally causes disease at that site. Our new variant might not be so choosy. It could bind to nerve tissue, the heart, skin, intestines or red blood cells, and cause severe, fatal disease as a consequence.

The future is statistical

For many scientists the future prospect for an influenza pandemic looks bleak. By a peculiar quirk of fate, this very morning I telephoned the responsible local authorities to report a dead duck that appeared on the lane where I live. In fact the duck looked very much as though it had been hit by a car, but it is entirely possible that the duck was dead from bird flu before it was run over. I was therefore contributing to the general anxiety about an avian influenza pandemic, although I behaved in a responsible way. But do I, as a doctor who deals with infectious diseases, believe that such a further pandemic is inevitable?

My answer is – maybe. The world is very different now from the situation in 1918. Then the globe was recovering from the war to end all wars. There was mass migration of demobilised soldiers to their native lands. We were totally unprepared for the disaster; the facilities to produce a vaccine were not available, nor were there effective drugs such as oseltamivir and zanamavir to treat the disease. The mode of transmission and therefore containment was poorly understood. We have all these advantages over the disease today. It might be argued that we are healthier, better nourished and more resistant to infectious disease nowadays, but the important caveat that pandemic influenza is very efficient at killing young, healthy people by 'cytokine storm' needs to be remembered.

There is one further reason that we might be spared the apparently inevitable Armageddon of pandemic avian influenza. The anxiety of scientists relies as much as anything on mathematics and statistics. In order for the virus to achieve its trick of transmitting between humans, it might only need to mutate by a very small amount by antigenic drift. Given the rate of mutation of influenza viruses, say the experts, such an event is inevitable. That may or may not be so, but that theory ignores the fact that such a mutation will not automatically ensure the catastrophic outcome so widely predicted. For a mutant to survive, it must, by the rules of natural selection, provide some evolutionary advantage to the virus. In other words, if the mutant capable of transmitting between humans arises in, say, wild ducks, it could simply die out, because it will be less effective at transmitting between ducks than the original strain was. Thus the emergence of the correct mutant is a necessary but insufficient requirement for disaster. We shall discuss the readiness of the world for the possibility of a worldwide pandemic in the final chapter.

The dangers we know

We should move on now from the theoretical future to the viruses that have caused epidemics in the past, or are continuing to do so. It would be impossible to include every virus responsible for every outbreak of human disease, or every one that has had any influence on human history. However, a number of viruses do demand further discussion – one that has been eradicated, two that almost were, and one that shows no such hope for the foreseeable future. The first category contains smallpox, the second polio and measles, and the final one HIV. The comparison between these diseases is fascinating for what they reveal about how humans have responded in recent history to such threats. These are very different viruses, with very different routes of transmission, different disease profiles and demographics. Nevertheless they tell us a great deal about what is happening to humankind, and where we are going in our response to epidemics.

Waclaw's story

Waclaw was 23. He had come from Poland to Britain to work as a labourer. In common with many of his countrymen, he liked to drink vodka. One evening the drink got the better of him and he fell into a canal. We encountered him a few days later when he developed a rash. Initially we thought he might have a condition called swimmer's itch – a parasite that lurks in water and can burrow under the skin and cause an intense reaction – but his dunk turned out to be a red herring.

There were a couple of features that did not fit the swimmer's itch hypothesis. One was the high fever and headache that he was enduring; the other were the tiny inflamed spots inside his cheeks, level with his back teeth. These are known as Koplik's spots. Waclaw had measles; he had never been vaccinated. He was lucky in that he developed none of the major complications of this disease: pneumonia, ear infections, even death. About half a million still die of measles worldwide every year.

Waclaw had almost certainly contracted the disease before he left Poland, where natural outbreaks of the disease still occur. There can be little doubt that the most effective intervention to control a viral epidemic is vaccination, and, despite the recent decline in uptake of the MMR vaccine, this potentially lethal illness remains rare in Britain, although a child died of measles in 2006.

Smallpox was finally eradicated by massive and concerted worldwide effort in 1977. The remaining episodes have been laboratory accidents, and sporadic reports from Africa that have turned out to be the related monkeypox. Polio is undergoing something of a resurgence, for reasons explained below. All of these diseases are eminently vaccine-preventable. By contrast HIV has cut monstrous swathes through nations, and remains incurable and without an effective vaccine. There were 26 million dead at the most recent count, with over 40 million infected worldwide.

Advances and limitations

We might pat ourselves on the back for the eradication of smallpox, apart from one major caveat. We could not repeat that feat today, at least not using the vaccine that was eventually used. The vaccine was developed, famously, by Jenner in the 18th century, from the related virus cowpox. He was not the first to experiment with cowpox, but he was the first to explore it systematically and to publish his results. There is absolutely no question in my mind that Jenner would have had his application to perform such experiments rejected by any modern ethics committee. And if he had managed to produce a vaccine, it would probably not have been licensed. That is perhaps understandable: there was at least one 20th-century smallpox outbreak where the mortality from the vaccine was greater than from the disease.

Further, there is some evidence that the vaccine that finally eradicated smallpox was actually contaminated by real smallpox. This was an accident, and almost certainly improved the efficacy of the vaccine, but it could not be repeated today. Our attitude to risk has changed. This is understandable given the falling mortality from infectious disease; whether our preciousness will remain justified in the face of other epidemics is yet to be seen.

Vaccines for polio would probably struggle to be licensed also; there were early disasters when the vaccine used in an attempt to prevent the disease actually caused it instead. However, there is a more distressing development in vaccination against this ancient enemy, the cause of infant paralysis, the disease that probably put America's wartime President Roosevelt in a wheelchair (although some say he was paralysed by another complication of an infection called Guillain-Barré). In some parts of the world people are rejecting the vaccine, driven by hysterical rumour-mongering and radicalised clerics preaching rabid anti-Western propaganda.

This has led to yet another human-made epidemic. Its epicentre has been the province of Kano, in Northern Nigeria. Salk's polio vaccination – administered by oral drops – has been refused by many thousands of Nigerians, in a trend which spread to Afghanistan and then Pakistan. More than 16 innocent bystander countries now have confirmed polio outbreaks, all neighbouring the countries where the vaccine has been rejected. The justification for rejecting it is that the West, in particular the US government, is supposed to have deliberately poisoned the vaccine with either HIV or a drug to suppress fertility among certain religious groups. The consequence of this superstitious drivel is that a disease on the very brink of annihilation is back with us again.

It is worth noting that smallpox was not eradicated by vaccinating every single individual in the whole world. That effect was obtained by an obsessive hunt for outbreaks and vaccinating those in the immediate vicinity. Wherever there was an outbreak, there was always the hazard that it could once again spread worldwide, unless each was properly dealt with. The same is true with polio. Every new case represents the continuing global presence of a disease which could so easily vanish into history. How sad it is that the original plan was to eradicate the illness by 2005.

For science and anti science

The ugly story described above represents something new and chilling in our struggle with epidemics. Since Pasteur finally and conclusively proved the germ theory of disease, replacing the fallacious doctrine of spontaneous generation, the trend throughout the world has been the suppression and cure of infectious diseases through science, experiment and proof. Most scientific progress, and the lead in disease control, has been from the West, often through the auspices of the WHO, with the explicit support of developing nations. Almost without exception, modern antibiotics, antivirals and vaccines have been invented in the developed nations of the West.

The rejection of polio vaccine in certain developing nations, and the drop in uptake of some vaccines like MMR in countries like Britain, represents something more than simply suspicion about science from the poorly educated and misguided. It represents a troubling trend in rejection of the values of the West, from both without and within. Of the rejection of polio vaccine by the ill-educated acolytes of bigoted clerics, and the rejection of MMR by supposedly educated and informed parents led by the discredited scientist Andrew Wakefield, the former is likely to have more impact while the latter is more distasteful.

Contrast the above with HIV, the virus against which we need a vaccine most urgently. This is proving almost impossible to develop. The virus is in many ways extraordinary, being like a snowflake. No two HIV viruses are ever identical, even if they come from the same individual. Add to this the fact that there is no comparable animal model of HIV infection, and some of the difficulties involved in developing a vaccine become apparent.

I have also heard the view put forward that the profit involved in long-term prescription of drugs that suppress HIV without curing it means that drug companies have little incentive to develop a vaccine. Whatever the truth, the inescapable fact is that it is proving extremely difficult to create one that works. We can add to this the change in the view concerning risk and ethics in drug and vaccine development. Jenner developed his vaccine with methods that seem impossibly hazardous by today's standards. Could you imagine a family doctor nowadays blithely inoculating a virus he fancied might prevent HIV into local children without permission?

It has been decreed that testing any drug or vaccine, whether for HIV or for any other illness, should be carried out using the same ethical standards in the developing world as would be applied in the West. Superficially this seems fair and reasonable, until you consider those 26 million deaths, those bald figures of incidence and mortality, and where they occur. HIV/AIDS is a quite different disease in most developing countries from the one we encounter in the West. At one extreme, in some countries it is even caused by a different virus – HIV-2 occurs in West Africa, and is not even susceptible to some of the drugs that are active against HIV-1. Because health care in many developing countries is rudimentary, HIV mortality is far higher even in the early stages of disease. This is not just a question of the availability of anti-HIV drugs. Even in the very early stages of infection, long before such drugs become necessary, the immunity of victims fails to recognise some common bacteria which are lethal if untreated. This is an inconvenience in Western countries, but kills elsewhere. Where the disease behaves so differently, does it make sense for us to fight it using the same tactics, effectively with one hand tied behind our backs?

I would argue that it might be prudent to rethink our nicety about such matters. I would also argue that the hesitancy of the West about taking desperate remedies for desperate times is part of the same collective failure of confidence in the values it represents. The decision not to apply different ethical standards to experimentation in the countries where the epidemic is felt at its most damaging is surely informed at least in part by the guilt the West feels about its colonialist, imperialist past. To me this makes no sense. Polio and smallpox have only been vanquished, or partly so, by bold strategies. The story of development of polio vaccine was not without its casualties. Atoning for the errors of the past is a poor tactic for tackling the problems of the present.

I shall conclude this chapter with a final thought about the relationship of humans to the world of viruses. One message of this chapter is that the notion of humans as a separate species with our own private set of genes is a bogus one. We stand in a constant genetic flux, where genes from viruses pass through all species, including us. This is an inevitable consequence of the origins and structure of life itself. These are not selfish genes; they are generous genes. All of us can make use of them. As we see in the next chapter, this is not a property confined to viruses.

CHAPTER 2

BACTERIA

I have long lost count of the patients I have seen with tuberculosis. One I remember most vividly is Gaynor. She was the third member of her family to contract the infection, and had developed symptoms in her lungs during early adolescence. The hormonal surges of that stage of development had two consequences for her. First, the disease is more likely to reactivate in puberty, as various sex steroids produced by the adrenals ebb and flow. Second, her mental state and compliance with the demands of her treatment were unstable and unreliable. Put simply, she was too bolshy to take her pills properly. Tuberculosis requires a minimum of six months continuous treatment. Gaynor intermittently refused to take her tablets.

If you were going to design an experiment where you wanted to ensure that resistance emerged in the tubercle bacillus, this would have been almost perfect. Sporadic treatment allows the bacterium an opportunity to ponder the problem of troublesome antibiotics at its leisure. We shall discuss the mechanics of bacterial resistance later, and of course bacteria do not actually 'ponder', but the terrible result for Gaynor was that each successive (and increasingly toxic) treatment failed, and she ended up with progressive destruction of her lungs from multi-drug resistant tuberculosis (MDR-TB). Eventually we had to resort to the kind of treatment that seems to belong more to the 19th century than the 21st: she had to have a lung completely removed. By the time this happened Gaynor was beyond adolescence, and viewed her misguided teenage rebellion with regret.

The disease we thought we had conquered

This is the disease that my parents' generation were told they would never encounter. It is now annually killing in the order of 2 to 3 million people worldwide, and has been declared a global emergency by the WHO. It would be deeply satisfying for the purposes of my theme to confirm one of the great theories about tuberculosis, that it is a disease of cattle and began to trouble humans when animal husbandry brought us into closer contact with such animals. Animal husbandry is one of the defining characteristics of modern humans; it would thus support the premise that it is our essential nature that makes us epidemics. However, the most recent evidence suggests that it happened the other way around, and we infected the poor cows.

Tuberculosis is the slow-motion epidemic. Its peaks and troughs can be measured in decades and centuries rather than months and years. There are a number of reasons for this. The bacillus grows slowly – it can take eight weeks to culture it in the laboratory, and it can incubate within the body for decades before causing symptoms. Like most epidemics, populations develop protection over time. The epidemic was declining in Europe before the advent of treatment and the imperfect BCG vaccine, and now 98 per cent of cases of tuberculosis occur in developing countries. Those countries lag behind Europe in the timing of their epidemic, which partly explains their higher incidence. However, this is yet another epidemic which persists for depressing reasons: poverty and failure of will.

Added to this equation is the evolving disaster of HIV/AIDS, which is particularly conducive to the development of tuberculosis. This combination has permitted the disease to transmit to the extent that one-third of the world's population is believed to be infected with the bacillus, and with the terrifying added complication that it is increasingly resistant to many drugs, as Gaynor discovered. Tuberculosis is also resurgent in the West now; the number of cases in Britain rises year on year. Much of this is the consequence of migrants arriving in the country with TB and/or HIV. This is the primary sense in which we *are* this epidemic; it is futile to think of controlling the disease in terms only of managing it in Western countries. The whole world is affected, and unless it is tackled in a global sense then all of us are at risk. No man is an island; we all share the risks of living on our tiny isolated planet.

Many of the major epidemics that have altered the course of human history have been caused by bacteria. Of my 'top ten' in the introduction, the Black Death, tuberculosis, the Great Pox, typhoid, cholera and typhus were all caused by these superficially simple single-celled organisms. Each of these has had incalculable impact, and Gaynor's disease continues to do so. Aside from their sheer numbers of victims, there is an extensive catalogue of major historical and artistic figures who have suffered and died from bacterial conditions. Tchaikovsky, for example, died of cholera. Mahler died of a heart infection following rheumatic fever as a child, as did Christopher Columbus (although some believe it was syphilis). Al Capone certainly died of syphilis, as Henry VIII may have; William McKinley (25th President of the United States) died of gangrene. There is an epic list of those who have died of tuberculosis, from the Brontë sisters to George Orwell.

Of course it is no surprise that so many famous names succumbed to bacterial diseases when they were the cause of so much mortality among the general populace. When formal records began to be collected in some countries, from about the mid-19th century, about one-third of deaths were caused by infection, and many of these would have been caused by bacteria.

The ubiquitous bacterium

Bacteria are everywhere, and we are made of them. We shall return to the most surprising aspect of that statement at the end of this chapter. However, the claim is true in a very straightforward sense, by simple weight of numbers. There are about ten times as many bacterial cells in a human body as there are human cells. The figures are in the order of 100 million million human cells in a human being, and 1,000 million million bacteria in his or her intestine. Bacteria comprise a lesser proportion of our body mass than these numbers might suggest, however, because they are smaller than human cells.

Before we proceed to examine the effects of the epidemics they have caused, it is important to understand what a bacterium actually is. For the sake of simplicity we shall define bacteria as packets of genetic information – DNA – contained within a single cell which usually has a wall of varying complexity. They are often capable of independent reproduction, unlike viruses, and they usually do so without sex by dividing into two identical offspring. They may live independently or be parasites upon other organisms. As forms of life they are massively diverse and widespread.

We probably know only a tiny fraction of the total that exist on the planet. Even in our own bodies there are many unidentified types; in our mouths alone probably only about half have been properly characterised. Extend this to more remote habitats – the sea, for instance – and the proportion that we know about falls to less than 1 per cent. We are constantly immersed in a teeming broth of bacteria. They are on our skin, in our hair, in our intestines in enormous numbers, on every surface imaginable. It would not really be labouring a point to claim that there is no such thing as a truly sterile environment, free from bacteria – except perhaps in the centre of a flame or other extreme heat source such as a volcano, and even this latter is a temporary state of affairs. Given the remarkable ability of bacteria to thrive in even the least promising of environments, it may seem surprising that diseases caused by them do not constantly threaten us and make us ill, and even threaten the very nature of humankind. In fact only a tiny proportion of the bacteria we encounter ever cause us harm.

The Great Plague

Unlike many of the other illnesses that form the essence of this book, I cannot describe a case of the most dramatic and catastrophic of the bacterial epidemics because I have never seen one. That is not to say that there are no longer people with the disease; it still crops up in Africa, South-East Asia, China and South America, and occasionally even the United States. This is the disease that wiped out between a third and a half of the population of Europe in the Middle Ages: the Great Plague, or the Black Death. It was an epidemic *par excellence.* In its classical form, as many will know, it is a bacterial infection transmitted to humans from the flea of the black rat. In its pneumonic form it is transmitted by inhalation of coughed-up infected droplets. We shall discuss how it arose, how it spread through populations, what people did to try to stop it, and why it disappeared. Could it ever come back?

First, though, a description of the illness itself. Unsurprisingly given the huge death toll from the scourge, there are many contemporary writings that eloquently evoke the horror of suffering from it. Pepys, Defoe, Boccaccio, Petrarch and Thucydides have all handed down to us their vivid accounts of what is generally assumed to be bubonic plague. We shall return to question that assumption; however, there is little doubt about the cause of the illness described by Boccaccio in the preface to

The Decameron. The earliest signs were ulcerating masses in the armpits and groins, these being the eponymous buboes. Black or livid purple blotches would then erupt rapidly through the body; hence the 'Black' Death. Modern medicine has a ready explanation for these discolourations. It is the failure of the blood to clot in the tiny vessels of the skin that causes haemorrhage and death of the tissues. It is a consequence of advanced septicaemia, and even with modern health care this condition has a high mortality. In the Middle Ages a disease that reached this stage would have been uniformly fatal. Doctors nowadays know it as disseminated intravascular coagulation, or DIC for short.

The condition of black or purple blotches on the skin shortly followed by death is by no means confined to the Black Death. There is a long list of causes, some infectious, others not. Septicaemia – overwhelming reproduction of bacteria in the blood stream – from many different organisms may lead to this terrifying conclusion. Possibly the most notorious arises from infection with *Neisseria meningitidis*, one of the most virulent causes of bacterial meningitis. There is a list of viruses that may have the same consequence, notably the dreaded viral haemorrhagic fevers like Lassa and Ebola. However, catastrophic infection with far less exotic agents can have identical consequences. Shock from blood loss and massive trauma may also lead to DIC. I am labouring this point because the classification of the Black Death of Europe of the Middle Ages as being exclusively due to *Yersinia pestis* has been questioned, as we shall see.

Should I encounter a case of a sick person with buboes in the armpits and groins I should probably have little difficulty (although great surprise and alarm) in establishing the cause. Even a milder case, with just the earlier symptoms of fever, chills and headache, should not necessarily delay diagnosis. I would be able to analyse specimens of tissue and blood in the laboratory and the characteristic features of the causative agent would soon reveal themselves. *Yersinia pestis* – unlike other more fastidious microbes such as the cause of Legionnaire's disease – is not a difficult organism to grow on ordinary Petri dishes, and its subsequent identification would not be challenging.

For this reason, as well as the facts that relatively straightforward antibiotics will cure the disease, and that there is a vaccine available, the chances of plague returning as an epidemic are slim indeed. We could cure and prevent it. However, we can do so because we stand upon the shoulders of great men. In this case that colossus is Alexandre Yersin (1863–1943), who isolated the bacillus which, since 1970, has borne his name, previously having been known as *Pasteurella*. Yersin demonstrated the plague bacillus in Hong Kong in 1894.

Yersin and after

Yersin was a trained Swiss-French microbiologist who had studied under another giant, Robert Koch. Yersin's involvement with diseases of infection arose through a dramatic accident. While performing a post-mortem on a patient in Paris who had died of rabies, he cut himself and injected himself with fluid from the still-infectious corpse. His likely death was prevented when he was inoculated with anti-rabies serum by another of the greats, Pierre-Paul-Émile Roux. From that moment Yersin devoted his life to the burgeoning field of microbiology.

He was sent to Hong Kong to investigate the plague ravaging that city, which had begun in China in 1860. His discovery of the plague bacillus – although almost simultaneously with a Japanese rival, Kitsasato – transformed the world. Identification of the disease in rats and their fleas allowed control of the source, and the days of the Great Plagues, still ravaging the Far East, were then numbered. The disease had to 'jump' to other rodents in the wild to survive, and it is from that source that most modern cases arise. The numbers in the modern world are not tiny – there were 10,000 cases per year in Vietnam during that country's disastrous war of the 1970s – but plague as an epidemic seems to have vanished. Yersin himself developed an anti-plague serum; nowadays treatment with commonplace antibiotics would readily yield a cure.

Contrast my privileged post-Yersin perspective with that of mediaeval physicians and priests who were faced with mass deaths from an unimaginable cause. These arose more than 500 years before the concept of disease caused by germs gained widespread acceptance. Several disastrous doctrines hampered the understanding of how illness in man and animals arose. One was that illness was divine retribution for unatoned sins. Another was the doctrine of spontaneous generation, which held that living organisms were capable of arising from inanimate matter – horseflies from dung, for example. It was to be many years before even the most primitive post-mortem was to be performed; given the dramatic sudden increase in mortality surrounding the first cases it is no surprise that those who passed for medical authorities at the time were reluctant to examine corpses. Most were buried in mass graves or even dumped in rivers.

In this state of ignorance, any series of mass deaths was likely to be attributed to the same cause. Thus it is by no means certain that all mortality from the plague years can now be attributed to *Yersinia pestis*. Attempts to identify the plague bacillus by recovering DNA from the mass graves of victims have met with variable success.

Death in Athens

Some historical plagues do not even match Boccaccio's classical description, judging by contemporary accounts. Thucydides described the Athenian plague which happened during the Peloponnesian war of the 5th century BC. A series of disastrous epidemics swept through Athens in those years, killing perhaps a third of the population. Accurate statistics from those times are understandably hard to come by; the Romans rarely counted beyond the number 600, a figure which also represented infinity. Buboes were not described as part of the syndrome. The symptoms were pain and difficulty in breathing, hoarseness, high fever, bruising of the skin and mental disturbance. A proportion, like Thucydides himself, recovered from the infection, unlike most victims of the bubonic plague, and these were capable of ministering to the sick. In other words, protective immunity had developed. Modern scholars and scientists still debate the cause of the Athenian plague. Typhus, say some; measles, complicated influenza, viral haemorrhagic fever, ergotism, say others.

Conversely and confusingly, the fact that the Athenian plague was not typical of bubonic plague does not rule Yersin's bacillus out of the equation. Indeed, it is this aspect of the study of diseases in humankind that makes it so fascinating and simultaneously troubling. It is a mistake to consider that both infectious agents and human populations are immutable. Infectious diseases may not be constant throughout history in their effects. This capacity to fluctuate depends upon at least two factors. One is the precise nature of the organism itself.

Yersinia pestis is an intracellular infection. That is, it causes its damage by gaining access to the inside of our cells. This is quite different from other types of infection – *Staphylococcus*, for example. The capacity to survive inside a cell is not present in all variants of the *Yersinia pestis* species. In other words it is entirely possible to culture a plague bacillus, identical in all other respects, that cannot cause illness. However, the properties of survival in cells, and causing illness, are transmissible.

Bacteria are able to pass genes among one another. They do so by a variety of mechanisms, in this example by exchanging packets of DNA. The resulting ability to survive inside a cell, or any other disease-causing property, is sometimes known as a virulence factor. The precise nature of the disease resulting from infection with a particular agent will depend on exactly which virulence factor is present. *Yersinia pestis* has many virulence factors, including one that prevents the blood clotting and thus leads to the famous black blotches. There is absolutely no reason that an ancient variety of *Yersinia* might not have had other virulence factors capable of causing the precise constellation of symptoms described by Thucydides. Indeed, the absence of one or more virulence factors might have conferred the higher likelihood of recovery. One of the features sometimes cited as a reason that bubonic plague was not a cause of the Athenian epidemic is the disappearance of the animals traditionally believed to carry the disease. One possible explanation is that this particular variant had virulence factors lethal to rats and rodents. This is one worrying aspect of the world of epidemics – we are constantly challenged by a moving target.

The second factor that may influence the progress and manifestations of an epidemic is the nature of the infected population. In its simplest form this just means the state of health and nutrition of the disease's victims, their level of overcrowding and the sophistication of public hygiene. In the ancient world, access to fresh produce would have been mostly seasonal; there would inevitably have been fluctuations in intake of vitamins vital for healthy response to infections. Vitamin C, found in fresh fruits and vegetables, for example, is not only vital for adequate disease resistance: a deficiency will cause defects in blood clotting that may compound the DIC we have already met in the Black Death.

In the context of the greatest epidemics of history, the Black Death, there are then a number of possible hypotheses, each of which if correct would have consequences for the possible evolution of new epidemics in modern times. The first is that all of the victims of the Black Death were genuinely infected with *Yersinia pestis*, whose virulence factors changed over time so that symptoms of the disease were not constant. Eventually it disappeared from Europe because it spontaneously downgraded its virulence. There are other examples of this phenomenon.

Streptococcus pyogenes was once the feared cause of rheumatic fever, with occasional consequent major damage to the heart. That bacterium, which remains common, appears to have spontaneously changed its virulence factors in recent times, making the once-common diagnosis of rheumatic fever relatively rare. The implication for us now is that any bacterium might equally spontaneously decide to upgrade its virulence and lead to an entirely new variety of illness.

The Black Death might have been entirely caused by Yersin's bacillus, but humankind evolved improved immunity to the infection. Eventually there would have been insufficient susceptible individuals for transmission to become possible, and the disease died out. In its simplest form this might mean that all susceptible individuals died. As we have said, statistics from antiquity are far from reliable, but there are certainly records from monasteries, for example, where every single inmate died. We might nervously infer from this that a new variety of epidemic might pursue the same course.

Run rabbit run

A possible and uncomfortable comparison might be myxomatosis in European rabbits, where the initial mortality rate was in the order of 99 per cent. The European rabbit is now recovering, some 50 years after myxomatosis was introduced to the continent from South America. There was, in fact, a very good reason that the rabbit population ultimately survived the myxomatosis epidemic, and one that potentially has consequences for humankind.

Myxomatosis spreads between rabbits by three routes – direct contact, fleas and mosquitoes. The most effective route, with the highest mortality, is via mosquitoes. In countries like Britain, where mosquitoes tend to vanish in the colder months, fleas and direct contact became more important. A few years after myxomatosis arrived in Britain, it was noticed that the rabbits had changed their behaviour. They had started to live outside their warrens, with less contact with other rabbits. Presumably the rabbits had not worked this out for themselves; there were, by chance, a few less sociable animals in any warren. They would previously have been at something of a disadvantage in terms of breeding, which most definitely requires contact with other rabbits. However, their solitary nature saved them when myxomatosis arrived. Thus a feature that was disadvantageous to the species in better times became a distinct survival advantage. It must be assumed that the tendency of rabbits to become solitary and live outside the warren is hard-wired into their genes, otherwise it would revert after a generation and the rabbits would once again become susceptible.

Resisting the Black Death

A disease with a mortality as high as the Black Death would almost certainly have selected out similar characteristics among humans. In other words we are living with the genetic, evolutionary consequences of exposure to this infectious agent of mass slaughter. Some of these might be variations in immunity that confer higher resistance to *Yersinia pestis*. Indeed, there is a hereditary defect in white blood cells which occurs in about 10 per cent of northern Europeans, which confers resistance to HIV. It is called the CCR5 delta-32 mutation. Some scientists have hypothesised that this protective mechanism which prevents the virus entering the cell arose as a consequence of the massive mortality associated with the plague. There is a major flaw to this argument: *Yersinia pestis* is a bacterium, HIV a virus. The delta-32 mutation provides no protection against bacterial infection. There is another possibility already referred to, which is that the condition known as the Black Death was actually a viral infection, or a series of epidemics of different diseases. For the purposes of this discussion, though, we shall stick to the conventionally held view that the plague was indeed caused by *Yersinia*.

As far as we can tell, humans have not developed any significant resistance to *Yersinia pestis* infection. The reasons the plague disappeared are controversial: some say it was the disappearance of the rats, others believe it was a downgrading of disease virulence. Nobody knows for certain, but untreated bubonic plague would kill you or me just as reliably as it ever did. This is identical to European rabbits and myxomatosis, where immunity barely seems to have emerged – the rabbits that survived by living outside their warrens remain as susceptible as ever to myxomatosis when summer, mosquito-borne outbreaks happen along. If this is so in humans, then it is even more likely that hard-wired behavioural characteristics survive among us, and that these characteristics determine some aspects of modern human behaviour.

What might such behaviour be? Of course this is highly speculative and not amenable to scientific proof; therefore in terms of pure science we ought to reject it. Nevertheless the possibilities of such speculation are tantalising. There are potential clues in contemporary writings. Possibly the most graphic comes from *The Decameron* by Boccaccio. This is a fictional account of some friends who escape the plague by holing up in a villa near Florence. The introduction to the work is not fictional, and records Boccaccio's own observations of humankind's mediaeval brush with Armageddon. In his account, written in 1370–71, one of the consequences of the plague was a collapse of what were considered appropriate morals of the time. Women of rank consorted with their servants and men of lower orders.

Could it be possible that human sexual behaviour changed, and permanently, with the dramatic evolutionary pressure of the plague years? Could the plague have induced hard-wired, genetically programmed promiscuity into humans? If that were the case, one might predict an explosion of sexually transmitted infection within European populations in the Middle Ages – an infection like, say, syphilis. That disease did indeed appear at the end of the 15th century, and, with a series of peaks and troughs, was not properly vanquished until the advent of penicillin in the 20th century. It is now beginning to trouble us again.

The great plagues had a colossal mortality: up to 90 per cent in some outbreaks, and an overall toll of about one-third of the population of Europe. There is no doubt that this had enormous effects on the social structure of European nations. It is no coincidence that many of the guilds of trades and crafts originated during this period. Skilled labourers found they were at a premium simply by virtue of their rarity, and were able to command higher wages and demand improved working conditions. This in turn led to the establishment of guilds of craftsmen: a sort of primitive trade unions, with the ability to demand higher fees. Professional standards were also established among these guilds. Thus was established an entirely new class: no longer of the clergy, or the nobility, or the peasantry; not feudal underlings, but a bourgeois middle class with some fledgling political independence.

From these small beginnings can be traced the emergence of a labour movement, of a politicised middle class, and the erosion of the authority of church and crown. The professional standards to which the guildsmen aspired ushered in new inventions, mechanisation, a sophistication of the tool-using trait that defines humankind. Thus can be traced the industrial revolution, democracy, the ascendancy of the West, capitalism and the modern world. Would it be too bold to trace the seeds of our eventual disastrous over-consumption of the world's resources, with the accumulation of our effluent in the atmosphere, back to the cataclysmic social consequences of the great plagues?

Choice and evolution

This, though, is not the only way in which infectious, epidemic bacterial diseases with high mortality have affected the evolution of humankind. To understand the full effect, some discussion of the nature of genetic heredity is required, and the manner by which all organisms exploit the world they inhabit.

Darwinian evolution operates by means of adaptation over generations into 'niches' where organisms may prosper and reproduce. These niches are defined by a series of more or less complex interacting features which limit or permit the ability of a species to inhabit them. In its simplest form some organisms, for example, will evolve to occupy a certain range of temperature. If weather patterns alter such that the temperature falls or rises outside the comfortable range for that species, then the organism concerned will have a 'choice'. It can either migrate to a region that satisfies its temperature range, or it can adapt its physiology so that it can continue to inhabit the altered environment. The second of these two options inevitably involves a change in the nature of the organism. When the conditions are persistent and severe enough, eventually this will result in the evolution of a genetically distinct organism. However, there may be another option, and one that some believe has had profound effects on human evolution.

Suppose our species of animal that lives in the zone of changing climate is not completely homogenous. The animals differ slightly from one another. Some are more 'fit' than others. It is an axiom of Darwinism that the fittest are more likely to survive into the next generation. Perhaps some animals have minor alterations to their physiology. One animal, through a minor mutation of genes, is slightly sweatier than the others. In a cool environment, this is a disadvantage because sweating is not a passive process; it consumes energy and loses precious fluid. However, as the temperature rises through climate change, this sweaty creature begins to achieve an advantage over its cooler, drier neighbours. Eventually, if the temperature rise persists, this characteristic means that the sweatier animal is more likely to reproduce and its characteristics will become more widespread through the species.

In the context of epidemics of infectious disease, the types of challenge may be far more severe and complex than a gradual increase in temperature. In consequence the types of adaptation required may be far more dramatic. In the example cited above, the characteristic of sweatiness was a relatively minor and benign disadvantage to the animal concerned. There are examples of more severe adaptations that have evolved within species in response to infection.

Safety in sickness

'Bad luck to the child whose brow is salty to the kiss, for he is cursed and soon must die.' This is an axiom taken from 18th-century German/Swiss medical literature. Excessive salt in the sweat is one diagnostic characteristic of one of the most common inherited disorders, cystic fibrosis. Cystic fibrosis was once believed to confer protection against typhoid and cholera. Tantalisingly in this example both cystic fibrosis and cholera have as their basis a defect in salt handling. It is now generally believed that typhoid and cholera were never sufficiently common to have produced a gene as widespread as the one that causes cystic fibrosis, which occurs in one in 22 Western Europeans. The current most convincing theory is that the cystic fibrosis gene confers resistance to the great scourge, the captain of the men of death, tuberculosis.

This is the phenomenon known as balanced polymorphism, where inherited, disease-causing traits are acquired as protection from infection. The best known is sickle-cell disease, which protects from malaria. Almost certainly there are very many others as yet unidentified. Tay Sachs disease, an extremely unpleasant condition characterised by inexorable mental and physical decline in childhood, may be another balanced polymorphism for resistance to tuberculosis.

Let us take this argument a stage further. Suppose you are playing poker with the devil. To retain your soul you must win a certain number of hands. The devil allows you one single advantage: you can always shuffle the cards. On these terms you would be sure to do the job thoroughly; if your opponent detects a pattern of recurring cards then your soul is in greater jeopardy. So it has been with our constant war of attrition with epidemics. Our capacity to survive as a species relies on our ability to shuffle the cards, to introduce a random element into the selection of our genes in the face of the constant challenge of infection. This happens through sex; every time we produce offspring we shuffle the genes for the succeeding generation.

This capacity for the introduction of random elements into a struggle would have two possible consequences. On the one hand it will result in the appearance and survival of more unpleasant mutations like those that cause sickle-cell disease and cystic fibrosis. The proof for this is that once the infectious challenge is removed, the 'defective' gene tends to disappear – sickle-cell disease among Americans of African origin is slowly disappearing in that almost malaria-free country. This capacity for gene-shuffling will result in a greater tendency to what we may call 'mutagenesis' as a characteristic in itself. In other words, a species is more likely to survive in the face of the challenge of serial epidemic infectious diseases if it has a greater capacity for genetic adaptability.

Included in this may be a greater tendency for gene disruption with severe consequences, up to and including cancers. There are indeed examples of genes that have a well-established tendency to mutagenesis with the consequent development of cancers. Probably the best known is the Philadelphia chromosome. Should you be unfortunate enough to inherit this gene, you will have a greater likelihood of developing certain kinds of leukaemia. Interestingly, there is accumulating evidence that the trigger required to activate the chromosome and cause its deadly effects is an infection itself. In this case it is a virus, the agent of glandular fever, Epstein Barr Virus.

We shall return to the subject of epidemics and cancer in Chapter 7. I introduce it here to demonstrate another sense in which we are epidemics – epidemic diseases like tuberculosis, plague and malaria create exactly the kind of evolutionary pressure that forces mutagenesis.

The modern plagues

The developed world is currently undergoing bacterial epidemics of quite another sort, with a totally different means of transmission. Aside from the worldwide pandemic of HIV/AIDS we are also witnessing a dramatic increase in the number of cases of sexually acquired infections, in the form of chlamydia, gonorrhoea, herpes and syphilis. In some senses we have been here before. Not for nothing is smallpox known as small. This was to distinguish it from the Great Pox. This was just one of the names given to the condition we now know as syphilis. It has also been known as the French disease and the

Neapolitan disease; it was almost 50 years after it arrived in Europe that the term 'syphilis' was first coined. However, modern physicians who see syphilis do so in an entirely different form from the mediaeval Great Pox, as this not uncommon brief history will illustrate.

Helen was expecting her first child in her mid-20s. She was entirely well. She had come into contact with the infection service in our hospital simply as a consequence of a routine blood test. As is standard in pregnancy she had been screened for the diseases of infection that would put her and her baby at risk. These include toxoplasmosis, rubella, cytomegalovirus, hepatitis B, HIV herpes and syphilis. She had a clean bill of health in every regard except one – the test for syphilis was reactive. At no stage had she had any suggestion that she might have contracted the disease; she had no symptoms. The diagnosis was shocking to her. Fortunately she had, on testing, no suggestion of any other sexually transmitted infection, and the disease appeared not to be active according to her blood tests.

Her treatment was straightforward. The cause of syphilis – *Treponema pallidum* – remains gratifyingly sensitive to Fleming's great discovery, penicillin. Treatment of infected mothers in pregnancy is vital, as the bacterium can transmit across the placenta and severely damage the baby. So long as the mother is not allergic to penicillin, eradicating the bacterium is straightforward. What was less straightforward for Helen was confronting her husband and unearthing how the sexually acquired infection had intruded into their world.

This is principally how the modern doctor encounters syphilis. The grotesque and disfiguring destruction of face, skin and bone described in medieval texts and pictured in contemporary engravings is never seen now. Nor do we see the gross mental disturbance known as 'general paralysis of the insane', or the bizarre stamping gait, where victims smash their feet to the ground like circus clowns, of the spinal condition known as *tabes dorsalis*. The principal reasons for this are implied by the above anecdote. Syphilis is diagnosed early, by blood testing, long before the symptoms manifest themselves. Furthermore it has been readily treatable since penicillin became widely available in the middle of the 20th century. In the pre-antibiotic era, the function of the physician presented with many illnesses of infection was simply to observe as the patient deteriorated. However, there is another reason. Syphilis simply is not the disease it used to be. It changed very early in its history in the West, and why that should be is a fascinating conundrum with implications for all epidemics.

History of a scourge

There is considerable debate about how and when syphilis first appeared in Europe. The most commonly held theory is that Columbus brought it back with him from his trip to the New World in 1492. Certainly it began to appear in Europe shortly after his return, but there is some suggestion from diseased skeletons dating from earlier periods that syphilis may have been present earlier than was previously thought. Confusion has arisen in part because the damage to tissues from syphilis may resemble that of leprosy, an infection with an ancient European pedigree. One theory holds that the disease evolved from similar non-sexually transmitted infections in children caused by almost identical bacteria. These are known as yaws, bejel and pinta, and they cause often highly disfiguring skin ulcers. Whatever the exact date and source, shortly after the epidemic arose in Europe something very strange happened to it.

When syphilis first explosively appeared on the scene it was the most horrific condition. Ulrich von Hutten himself suffered from it, and recorded this account in 1519 in *A Treatise on the French Disease:*

> truly when it first began, it was so horrible to behold ... They had Boils that stood out like Acorns, from whence issued such filthy stinking Matter (pus), that whosoever came within the Scent, believed himself infected. The Colour of these was of a dark Green and the very Aspect as shocking as the pain itself, which yet was as if the Sick had laid upon a fire.

Contrast this experience with that of Helen, who only found out she had syphilis through a blood test. Indeed, most of the modern syphilis epidemics have been detected by the same method, the sufferers almost invariably having little or nothing in the way of symptoms.

So what happened to the disease to make it so different, such that 'one would scarce think the Disease that now reigneth to be of the same kind', in von Hutten's own words? The natural history of infection with this bacterium is that it passes through a primary stage – usually a painless ulcer on the genitals – to a secondary, symptomatic phase, before a latent period in which very little happens. Finally, in about a third of sufferers the disease reactivates. Patches of inflammation may appear more or less anywhere on the body; this is known as the tertiary or late stage. Sometimes reactivation occurs with a vengeance, destroying brain, heart, nerve and bone. This is sometimes known as quaternary syphilis, and this is the stage that kills.

Von Hutten's illness that was 'horrible to behold' was at the secondary stage. Secondary syphilis nowadays, when seen, is characterised by a mild rash but little in the way of symptoms. There may be a headache, swollen glands and runny nose, but there is almost never skin breakdown or boils; bone ache is usually trivial. It is barely 'as if the Sick had laid upon a fire'.

Why did syphilis change so much? One possibility is that natural immunity arose among the newly infected population. There is an objection to this: it happened too quickly. Some contemporary writers documented the extreme variants of secondary syphilis becoming more rare after only five to seven years; and this in a disease which generally does not kill in the secondary stage. This is far too short a time for generalised immunity to a completely new epidemic to arise. Besides, the proportion of untreated people who progress to the potentially lethal late tertiary and quaternary stages has not changed, from about a third. And yet by the mid-16th century the real venom had passed from the epidemic.

Looked at from a different perspective, though, there is a perfectly plausible explanation of how evolution may have taken a hand. Answer these questions: if you had to choose someone for a night of passion, would you pick an apparently healthy person with a rash only barely visible, or someone covered with stinking green boils the size of acorns who cries out in agony every few moments? When are people more likely to feel like sex – when they have a slight runny nose, or when they have bone pain so agonising that they can barely lie down? The question is barely worth asking, but has a clear consequence. Syphilis, unless in pregnancy, is only infectious in the primary and secondary stages. Thus there would be clear selection pressure *on the syphilis bacterium itself* for organisms that caused milder disease. Without sex the bacterium could not transmit and survive; variants that made their victims physically repulsive would slowly have vanished.

For the purposes of modern syphilis epidemics, this hypothesis has an important consequence. Ready, easy treatment has meant that syphilis has changed from being a common disease to a rare one. The selection pressure is in favour of the bacterium causing symptomless disease in its primary and secondary infectious stages, and this has been accelerated by the availability of safe and effective treatment. The late stage – the fatal one – is not infectious, and the bacterium is no longer under selection pressure. We are thus in a 'silent' epidemic of symptomless syphilis, which if undiagnosed may emerge many years later as fatal late disease. Thus humans are responsible for the nature of the current epidemic, which has seen a 1,000 per cent increase in new diagnoses of syphilis in the United Kingdom. This has almost entirely been an asymptomatic disease, diagnosed by blood tests in sexual health clinics.

Our friends the microbes

Early in this chapter I mentioned the astonishing outnumbering of human cells by bacterial cells within our bodies. It would be surprising if this mass occupation of our bodies was accidental and of no use to us. What is more surprising is how much we depend upon this epidemic of microbes that infests us. They are not simply passengers; they do a great deal of work on our behalf. While it is possible to survive without intestinal flora, it is considerably more difficult.

Their most obvious and well-known function is to digest food for us. They metabolise otherwise indigestible carbohydrates into usable sugars and fatty acids. They also perform a 'probiotic' function, resisting invasion by their other more dangerous cousins. A faintly repulsive example of this arises from the dangerous disease caused by *Clostridium difficile*. This bacterium can colonise the intestines of people who have been given antibiotics, usually in hospital. In extreme cases occasionally an attempt is made to restore the normal, probiotic flora (the normal healthy bacteria which line the intestine), using 'donor stool'.

Our intestinal bacteria perform other, more complex functions. Some people may owe their very existence to the capacity of bacteria to change the structure of hormones. If your mother was taking the contraceptive pill and also took antibiotics, the disruption to her intestinal flora might have meant that the pill was inactivated by the new bacteria which took their place.

Some bacteria metabolise sex steroids, and to our benefit. It would barely be stretching a point to talk about the microbes in our bodies as a separate organ. They perform a multitude of roles, on which we rely without thought, much like the functions of our lungs or kidneys. The simple fact is that the huge majority of the many species with which we share our lives cause us no problems whatsoever; in fact quite the reverse.

The colonisation of our bodies by these huge numbers of microorganisms poses a question about both us and them. The difference between bacteria that make us ill and bacteria that work for us may be tiny indeed. There is a dangerous bug called *E. Coli* 0157 which can cause epidemics of severe diarrhoea and kidney failure; it is only very slightly different from the billions of helpful *E. Coli* which usefully line our intestines. Why do we tolerate them, and how do we know which are the right ones for us?

The answer seems to be a remarkable property of bacteria, and one that we simply had not suspected until very recently. This property makes them much more like us than we had previously thought. Put simply, bacteria can communicate. In the real world, they do not live in isolated pure colonies of identical cells of the sort that are traditionally studied in laboratories. They live, cooperatively or in competition, in complex ecosystems where some provide food for others, or create oxygen-starved pockets where bacteria that are killed by oxygen may thrive, or attempt to kill rivals. These are called biofilms, and they occur almost everywhere in nature. Communication between them is carried out by hormones, very similar to our own, and these chemicals transmit signals to other bacteria of the same and of different species. They also transmit signals to us; 'healthy' bacteria signalling their benevolence, dangerous ones like *E. Coli* 0157 sending a malign message directly to our own hormones, which triggers the illness. This is quite different from a bacterium producing a poison, first because the great majority of the signals are the benign sort which 'calm' our immune cells and request a state of tolerance, and second because the dangerous signal is in itself harmless, but is directed at our own hormones, and causes us to do the damage to ourselves.

This property of bacterial communication is known as quorum sensing, because the signal is not produced until enough bacteria have amassed, exactly like a board meeting, where a 'quorum' of sufficient individuals is required before a decision can be taken. We are thus composed of bacteria by mutual consent. One consequence of the hormone signals that the bacteria send is that our intestinal cells 'feed' them with the right sort of sugars. Looked at obliquely you could almost argue that we are being 'farmed' by bacteria, in the sense that they tell us to provide food, and like dairy cows, we oblige. If the colonisation of our intestines is deficient, we become susceptible to a variety of diseases. On the other hand, some disease-causing bacteria exploit our tolerance to their benign cousins by mimicking their signals and behaviour to invade. Thus we are susceptible to disease because of our reliance on the bacteria that make us. If we did not need them, we would not suffer intestinal diseases like typhoid and dysentery. Thus we *are* epidemics.

We are bacteria

So far this chapter has concentrated on the effects of bacterial infections on individuals and humankind in general. There is no question that such infections have had immeasurable impact on our evolution as a species. There is, though, an even more startling observation to be made about evolution and bacteria. In the chapter on viruses I mentioned the large proportion of our genes that clearly arose from viral infection. Precisely the same is true of bacteria. Some of our genes, and whole building blocks of our cells, are composed of bacteria. This is not just true of all animals, it is also true of plants. To this extent it is less specific and defining of humanity than the viruses discussed in Chapter 1. Nevertheless it remains true that we are bacteria to a degree, and that our evolution was driven by an ancient epidemic that has continuing consequences.

Contained within every one of our cells is a small furnace, or more exactly several. They are the mitochondria. They produce energy within cells; they also produce toxic products. The mitochondrion has a number of properties that mark it out from other animal cell fragments. Firstly, it does not divide like animal cells, it divides like bacteria, in a process called binary fission. Mitochondrial membranes are different from the membranes of other animal cells, resembling bacteria more than animals. They contain their own ribosomes, which are the protein factories of cells. Most importantly of all they have their own genes. These genes are definitely not of animal origin.

So what is a mitochondrion, and where did it come from? Almost certainly they were once bacteria, or organisms very like them. At some unimaginably distant moment in the past they invaded a different type of cell, much like an amoeba. It is likely in that 'epidemic' that the vast majority of victims died. However, some of the amoebae then developed a tolerance for the invader, and then even a dependence. This has been demonstrated in modern experiments which have sought to reproduce that long-ago event. Amoebae can be artificially infected with similar bacteria in the laboratory. Initially, most die but a few survive and can reproduce. Eventually the amoebae become reliant on their bacterial contents, to the extent that they cannot survive when the bacteria are killed with selective antibiotics.

Now comes the really astounding part. Some of the genes of the invading bacterium and some of the genes of the amoeba have swapped. Mitochondrial genes contain genes that arose in humans, and human genes contain mitochondrial genes. This step – the exchange of DNA – was almost certainly an evolutionary necessity in order for the invaded cell to control its new guest. The mitochondrion no longer has a complete set of genes. It can no longer reproduce independently, and some regulatory genes are contained within the nucleus of the cell. In other words the tenant has handed over some aspects of its own regulation to its landlord. An organism which has within it a bacterium capable of unregulated reproduction is in dire straits – the invader will simply consume all the available nutrients, even if it produces no toxins. Therefore the amoeba that had the capacity to exchange DNA and regulatory genes with its invader would have been the variant that survived.

Competence

Contained within our ancestry, then, is a vital property, which is widespread among other organisms. Among bacteria it is referred to as 'competence'. This means the capacity to transmit and acquire genetic material from other organisms and even other species. The bacteria known as streptococci are especially 'competent'. It is not a property that has traditionally been ascribed to higher organisms like humans, at least in this strict scientific sense. It has usually been accepted that new genes are acquired in humans and other higher animals through sex, and, slowly through mutation. However, competence must have been present in the ancestry of animals that contain mitochondria (and plants that contain their equivalent, the chloroplasts), in order for regulatory genes to be shuffled around between host and victim.

You may think this is a dry and academic point to be making. If you consider the evidence presented in Chapter 1 on viruses, that an amazing 45 per cent of our genes are derived from so-called mobile genetic elements, then you might revise that view. Those mobile elements are of non-human origin, effectively viruses and bacteria. Without the bacterial property of 'competence' we could never have evolved. We are epidemics.

As I have said, the same has occurred in reverse, and mitochondria contain genes from their hosts. The consequence of this exchange of genes supports the underlying theme of this book, which is that humans are composed of infectious material, and are epidemics. In the context of this bacterial invasion this is true at multiple levels. We contain bacteria within our cells. Some of our genes are of bacterial origin. We have relied on a property peculiar to bacteria – competence – to permit our evolution to proceed.

The knowledge that not only have we co-evolved with infections, we *are* them, adds weight to the suggestion that we might find useful chemicals to fight infection within ourselves. Such speculation is not altogether new; in the chapter on viruses the chemical interferon is discussed. This is a protein produced by cells to fight certain kinds of infection, particularly viruses. It might be reasonable to expect that the same principle applies to bacteria.

Such is the case. It has long been known that human secretions like tears and saliva are far more complex fluids than simple salt water and mucus. Both contain many different chemicals of human origin, to the extent that many diseases can be readily diagnosed by testing these fluids for antibodies – HIV, for example, or measles. Contained within these fluids are also substances that are toxic to bacteria. They are surprisingly simple in structure – usually very short proteins – but deadly to the germs that threaten us. They are spears and bows and arrows rather than the nuclear strike of antibiotics, but none the less effective for that.

They go by a number of names, defensins and cationic antimicrobial peptides being the commonest. They are very particular to individual species, such that human defensins are quite different from even those of our closest evolutionary relatives. They are present in just about all tissues, including lungs, bladders, guts and skin. To date, bacteria simply seem incapable of developing resistance to them. They are also active against parasites and viruses. They seem to work by 'short-circuiting' bacteria. Our cells have no real difference in electrical charge between the inside and outside of the cell membrane, whereas bacterial cells do. Defensins slip themselves into the bacterial membrane and use the charge to kill the bug. You might not be surprised to learn that these compounds are proving to be of considerable interest to pharmaceutical companies. A naturally occurring (and therefore non-toxic) human substance that kills bugs but not people and seems to generate no resistance seems almost too good to be true.

The great bacterial epidemics of plague, tuberculosis and syphilis have thus shaped our destinies as humans, while our genetic make-up has been at least in part shaped by our immersion in the world of bacteria. As we have also seen, we are to a large degree composed of bacteria. We shall now move on to a different group of organisms, which have also shaped us to a greater or lesser degree. These are the parasites.

CHAPTER 3

PARASITES

The position of parasites in the league table of dangerous epidemics is principally maintained by a single disease. That disease is malaria, and it is one of the world's biggest infectious killers. We generally think of parasitic diseases as being confined to tropical countries. In Britain, for example, serious parasitic disease is encountered so rarely that there is only a single consultant parasitologist employed by the entire National Health Service. There are, though, many parasites that can cause epidemics in humans even in temperate countries. Pinworm, a relatively harmless roundworm which causes intense itching around the anus, is said to affect 42 million in the United States alone. As we shall see, parasitic infections are so widespread and common that we might consider them 'normal'.

Parasites are more complex organisms than the other causes of epidemics discussed in this book. For this reason they are bigger, sometimes even visible to the naked eye. Sometimes they are so big that their sheer bulk is the cause of disease, obstructing channels and vessels or squashing healthy tissue. Such is the case with the liver flukes, for instance, which may cause jaundice by obstructing the bile duct which drains the liver. They may be so big that they cause illness by successfully competing for body nutrients. Although, like viruses, they are unable to complete their life cycles and reproduce independently, they differ in that they have complete internal structures that can perform many of their necessary functions. They can, for instance, produce energy and enzymes for themselves. Viruses cannot do this, they have to hijack the cells of their hosts for these functions.

Like bacteria (but unlike viruses), parasites have cell walls, but these are often more complex than those of the simpler organisms. In at least one example, sleeping sickness, the cell wall performs an act of master disguise: it sheds and replaces part of its outer coat in serial fashion to evade the surveillance of white blood cells.

Parasites are generally more complex than bacteria in their life cycles. Bacteria reproduce asexually, by dividing into two identical offspring. Parasites may have two parts to this process, and this is where their requirement for hosts derives. Malaria, for instance, reproduces asexually by division at one stage of its life (in the victim) and sexually at another, by producing sperm and ova – in the mosquito. Both stages are vital for the parasite to survive, and thus malaria actually requires two hosts, although the mosquito is more commonly known as the *vector*. Parasites may have free-living forms, often in water, which may be infectious, but they cannot complete their entire life cycles in that state.

The complexity of their life cycles and of their structures is vital in their capacity to cause epidemics and to evade our attempts to control them. Malaria control requires both treatment of the victims and control of vectors. The complexity of their cell walls makes it harder to devise drugs that are toxic to the parasites but safe for us. Indeed, until recently, the treatments for two parasitic infections – sleeping sickness and loaiasis – were not much less dangerous than the diseases themselves.

I do not know of a stranger case of contracting malaria than the story that follows. I have altered one or two key facts to protect identities, but the story is essentially true.

Janet's story

People who are brought up in malarial areas are often reluctant to take prophylactic tablets to prevent the condition when they return home. This, then, is the story of one of those and the consequences of her foolhardiness. Janet had been brought up in southern Africa. She had had malaria repeatedly as a child, and thought herself more or less immune. Immunity to malaria can occur, but it tends to be short-lived and to wane rapidly once people are no longer exposed. When Janet married she was keen to show her new husband the countries of her childhood. The pair of them undertook a two-month honeymoon tour of most of the countries of southern Africa. Janet did not take any malarial prophylaxis at all.

On the way back to London she and her husband stopped in Italy, where she began to feel ill. She had fevers and felt sick.

Her concerned husband took her to the local hospital. The staff decided she had a touch of traveller's diarrhoea – exposure to the local strains of bacteria to which her intestine was not acclimatised – and simply gave her some fluid through a drip before letting her go back to her hotel.

The next stage of the journey was to London. By the time Janet landed at Gatwick she felt dreadful. She had high fevers, headache and began to seem confused to her husband. He sought help at the airport. She was taken to the local hospital, whose staff almost immediately diagnosed malaria. In fact not only did they diagnose malaria, they diagnosed it in spades. Serious malaria is defined as having more than 2 per cent of the red blood cells containing the parasite. More than 40 per cent of Janet's were infected, a state of affairs that is not really compatible with life. She was transferred to the intensive care unit, and the advice of infectious disease physicians was sought. She was desperately ill for a few days, but with a combination of the skill of the doctors and a following wind of good luck she survived. Within ten days she was home.

The doctor who saw her at her subsequent out-patients appointment was pleased to see that she had fully recovered, but noticed her emotional distress. She handed him a letter she had received from the hospital in Italy where she had been treated for traveller's diarrhoea. The cause of her distress became immediately apparent. The letter said that the Italian doctor who had treated her was dead. He had developed a feverish illness a few days after Janet had left. Malaria has been unknown in that part of Italy for many years, and so the diagnosis was not made until too late – at post-mortem, in fact. It transpired that while he had been setting up the drip for Janet's infusion of saline, he had managed to jab himself with the needle contaminated with her blood. This is known as a needlestick injury: they are common in medical practice, and more commonly transmit hepatitis B, C and HIV. This poor doctor had inoculated himself with blood teeming with malaria parasites. It was simply his bad luck that he had not made an accurate diagnosis on Janet himself. He paid for this error with his life.

Malaria and us

The origin of malaria almost certainly represents our own evolutionary origins. The four main causes of human malaria – *Plasmodium falciparum, vivax, malariae* and *ovale* – are confined to humans. There are, though, almost identical organisms that cause very similar illnesses in the great apes. Almost certainly the parasite evolved with primates and co-evolved with humanity. This is reflected in the fact that accounts of malaria can be found in the very earliest writings of our species, and without doubt malaria has always been with us. Shakespeare refers to it – as 'the ague' – and it has been described by Chaucer, Hippocrates and Homer. The earliest known written reference is from the Chinese Nei Ching Canon of Medicine of 1700 BC; there is an almost equally ancient reference in the Ebers papyrus of 1570 BC.

Malaria remains a killer of pandemic proportions in the developing world, with 300 million cases per year and 1–2 million deaths, many of them children. However, it once caused huge numbers of cases in the West, with 500,000 cases annually in the

United States alone. Indeed, the Centers for Disease Control in Atlanta, Georgia, where data on infectious diseases are collated and plans for control hatched, began their life as the Office of Malaria Control. In Europe the disease extended as far north as England, and was endemic in undrained marshlands such as the Lincolnshire fens until relatively recently. Oliver Cromwell, a fensman himself, is said to have died of the disease. Malaria remains so common in many countries that it has forced human evolution down a tricky and dangerous path.

Teri's story

Teri was from a black African family; her great-grandparents migrated to the south-west of England. I met her when I was a junior doctor working in Bristol. She was then 23. She was admitted to our hospital with agonising pain in her bones which required morphine, one of the most powerful painkillers available, as well as an intravenous drip of saline and an oxygen mask. Her pain was caused by obstruction to her blood vessels. She also lacked a spleen; recurrent and very painful blockages to bloodflow in that organ had caused it to die, quite literally, inside her.

On this occasion we were able to control her symptoms until the concentration of oxygen in her blood rose and the blockages cleared. In the future she would not be so fortunate. This unpleasant and relatively common condition is associated with tragically early death. Low oxygen in Teri's blood would lead to distortion in her red blood cells, which would stick together and jam up her circulation. The starved tissues would increase her requirement for oxygen, and compounded by dehydration, a vicious circle would develop. She had inherited a defect in the construction of her blood cells which made them fold and become sticky. Under the microscope the cells appear to be curved and shaped like sickles, quite unlike the regular doughnut shapes of healthy red blood cells. This is how Teri's condition got its name – as I am sure you have guessed, this is sickle-cell disease.

At first it might seem bizarre that such an unpleasant condition is so common in some populations of the world. In Uganda, for instance, 46 per cent of the population carry one of the two genes required for sickle-cell anaemia to develop; these are known as carriers, or sickle-cell trait, because they generally do not suffer the consequences of abnormal blood cell shape. Two copies of the gene – one derived from each parent – are required to cause the full-blown disease. One-quarter of all offspring where both parents are carriers might be expected to inherit both genes and thus develop symptoms like Teri's. Because the illness carries a high mortality in young life, the number of people with actual sickle-cell anaemia is far lower than might be expected, the reality in Uganda being in the order of 2 per cent. Both figures – numbers of carriers and people with disease – fall significantly in populations who have migrated away from the regions of their ancestry. African-Americans, for example, have a sickle carrier prevalence of only 8 per cent, with only 0.25 per cent suffering the illness. The difference between the populations is their exposure to one infectious disease in particular – malaria.

The malaria parasite needs to enter human red blood cells to complete its life cycle and survive. In doing so, it causes illness by rupturing the cells and causing them to 'stick' in blood vessels, in a way not unlike sickle-cell anaemia. The abnormal red blood cells of sickle-cell disease deny the parasite entry, and even the state of being a carrier of the sickle-cell trait provides some protection from invasion by the deadly protozoon. The gene for sickle-cell disease persists for that reason. Malaria is a disease with a high mortality. Even apparently severe disadvantages as sickle-cell disease may be 'tolerated' by evolution to protect against it. This is balanced polymorphism; we have encountered it already in tuberculosis and cystic fibrosis.

Knowledge of the historical development of the condition was of cold comfort to Teri, living in the malaria-free south-west of England. Among human populations with a high incidence of malaria, this genetic defect survives; however, over generations living in countries like Britain and the United States, the advantage of having the gene disappears, and in fact becomes a pure disadvantage. Thus it slowly vanishes. Teri's genetic blueprint, the very essence of her being and the ultimate cause of her premature death, derives from epidemic infectious disease. This is shared by huge numbers of people worldwide, and it is worth noting that even the apparently harmless carrier state of sickle-cell trait can end in severe and symptomatic disease in the context of severe dehydration, exposure to high altitude or lung infection.

Balanced polymorphism

There are certainly other examples of balanced polymorphism that have probably evolved as a consequence of the exposure of humans to other infectious epidemics. The sickle-cell/malaria example is the most well known, and broadly accepted by scientists. There are other similar defects related to other populations – thalassaemia, for instance, among Mediterranean peoples – which share the same malarial origins. However, as was discussed in the chapter concerning bacteria, there is accumulating evidence for others. Indeed, there are many who believe that a large number of severe inherited diseases have arisen as protective mechanisms against infectious disease. In this sense, then, humans are epidemics only indirectly. Some of our genetic make-up is the reflection of our encounters with epidemics. Furthermore, the ultimate fatal destiny of those who die young from inherited diseases like Tay-Sachs and cystic fibrosis is dictated by our species' struggles with epidemics.

The effects of parasitic infection in the form of balanced polymorphism are thus a rather indirect if severe influence on humankind. Human geopolitical history has been dictated in a far more direct way by other parasites, both including and excluding malaria. For millennia they have decided where we live, or more accurately where we cannot live. Some regions of the globe have historically been rendered uninhabitable for humans by the burden of parasitic disease. Sleeping sickness is an excellent example, as is onchocerciasis, also known as river blindness.

The bugs drive us out

At first sight it may not seem obvious that parasitic illnesses should govern where humans may thrive or not thrive any more than any other disease of infection, be it from viruses, bacteria or fungi. Sleeping sickness, for example, is not entirely dissimilar in its symptoms to many other chronic infections such as tuberculosis; lassitude, fever, malaise and weight loss predominate in both. The crucial difference is the route of transmission and the source of the diseases in the natural world.

Humans transmit tuberculosis to other humans. In other words, wherever you are in the world, if you encounter an infected and contagious individual, your chances of becoming infected rely solely on luck. Of course if you are in a region where a very high proportion of the people are infected then your risk increases, but it does not matter precisely where in the world the encounter happens. Sleeping sickness, by contrast, is a disease of domestic cattle and humans limited to particular geographical regions by its vector. The natural reservoir of *Typanosoma brucei var. Rhodesiense*, the agent of the more severe variant of the disease, is wild antelope, who appear to suffer no harm from harbouring it. The parasite is transmitted to humans through the bite of tsetse flies of the genus *Glossina*. This fly is limited in its distribution by climate. Thus in order for sleeping sickness to be endemic in a region, a combination of suitable climate, presence of the fly and domestic animals such as cattle is required.

Where this lethal constellation arises the consequences can be disastrous. This disease was once the scourge of central and eastern Africa. The population of southern Uganda fell by a third in less than 20 years after the disease appeared there in an epidemic of 1896. Sleeping sickness has almost certainly been endemic in western Africa for many generations, and indeed whole tracts of land were once rendered uninhabitable, at least for herdsmen and their cattle, by this vicious infection. The situation has improved in recent years, through the cunning and artifice of man in controlling the fly. For some reason tsetses are attracted to stripes of blue and black; traps can be tailored from pyramids of such coloured cloth and because the fly lays a single egg, it can virtually be eradicated by such simple techniques.

The disease requires specific ecological conditions, and is thus confined to particular geographical areas. This is not to say that the distribution of sleeping sickness has not been affected by human intervention and migration. Indeed, many believe that the British explorer Henry Morton Stanley may have helped to spread the illness along the Congo basin while attempting to rescue a provincial governor of Southern Sudan called Eduard Schnitzer from the clutches of Islamic rebels. This expedition began in 1887 and involved 1,500 men moving through the rainforests to Lake Victoria; some say the epidemic that struck southern Uganda so brutally a few years later came with Stanley's men. With supreme irony when Stanley came upon Schnitzer he initially refused to be rescued, and indeed eventually returned to the Sudan where he was killed in 1892. Hundreds had died trying to rescue him.

This poignant and colourful story reflects much of the modern experience of sleeping sickness, and its migration along routes taken by the colonial invaders of the last 150 years. There is an irony here: the white settlers and explorers who tried to open up the heart of Africa to exploit its natural resources simultaneously closed them down by spreading sleeping sickness to new areas. Previously it had been confined by the static cultural traditions of the original inhabitants. These recent perturbations of a previously more stable and harmonious balance between humans and disease have clearly significantly altered the situation, and the effects of this derangement persist to this day.

There are plenty of articles to be found in the medical and historical academic literature that point a steady finger of blame at European white settlers for the resurgence of sleeping sickness in the early 20th century. This accusation may or may not be accurate, but we could argue that those settlers behaved precisely like the tsetse fly. We can hardly blame the flies; there is no point in blaming an animal for behaving like an animal. When their natural sources of blood are scarce, tsetses will seek out other sources. In the late 19th and early 20th centuries a wave of a viral illness called rinderpest swept Africa. Cattle and wild animals died in droves. The blood-feeding tsetse was forced to hunt further afield. Coincidentally European explorers like Stanley were penetrating the continent at the same time. We could go on to argue that those explorers were the vanguard of a migration from Europe escaping sudden massive over-population, and that they were responding to the same biological needs as tsetse flies.

Mary's story

Mary was a 20-year-old trainee nurse, recently arrived from Nigeria, who came to our clinic with intense itching of the skin. She had been referred to our department because her family doctor felt she might have an exotic infection from her country of origin. His surmise was supported by some basic blood tests; her white cell count was markedly abnormal. In particular, she had a significant excess of cells called eosinophils, often a marker of infection with parasites.

When we examined her it was hard not to spot the evidence of her distress; her skin was scarred and scratched from frequent assault by her fingernails. She was also covered in multiple tiny bumps, about the size of lentils. We strongly suspected onchocerciasis. Diagnosis is traditionally made by taking snips of skin and putting them to soak in saline for a period. It is then possible to see the tiny migrating worm under the microscope. To ensure not to immobilise the teeming hordes the snips must be taken, cruelly, without anaesthetic. We elected not to put Mary through this ordeal. The diagnosis may also be made with blood tests, and there is a safe and reliable treatment. The almost mediaeval practice of snipping live skin from an unanaesthetised patient is probably best reserved for when proof is elusive.

Mary was indeed suffering from onchocerciasis. This is caused by a parasite called *Onchocerca volvulus*, which can lead to a condition called river blindness, should the worm migrate to the eyes and die there. It is transmitted by the bite of the blackfly. Unlike sleeping sickness, humans are the only known reservoir of *Onchocerca*. As its name suggests it is a disease of riverine areas, and the fly prefers fast-flowing water. Such regions are attractive for settlement as they are fertile. It is endemic in 36 nations worldwide, affecting 18 million people, principally in Africa, although it also occurs in Latin America, probably carried into that continent by the slave trade.

Itching and blindness

Although the illness does not kill people in itself, the infection reduces the host's immunity and resistance to other diseases. This results in an estimated reduction in life expectancy of 13 years. It causes blindness only in a minority of infected individuals. However, its principal symptom is agonising and persistent itching, which can result in disfiguring scarring of the skin. People do not like living in areas afflicted by river blindness, for reasons that must now be obvious. This naturally has wide-reaching economic effects, closing down otherwise fertile productive regions.

Larvicides, which kill the blackfly in its larval form, and a drug called ivermectin which treats the infection and thus the capacity of the victim to transmit it, have been the key to controlling river blindness. Since the 1970s 25 million hectares of previously abandoned land in West Africa alone have been opened up for agriculture by control of river blindness. This land is estimated to be capable of feeding 17 million people long-term. These are not trivial numbers, and the economics of entire nations like Nigeria are affected by such infestations.

To state that the entire geographical distribution of humankind is dictated by the relative presence or absence of such parasites is clearly an exaggeration. Nevertheless parasitic infection still exacts an enormous toll on human welfare. In the developing world parasites are extremely common. The bald figures speak for themselves. We could almost draw the conclusion that the 'natural' state for humankind is to harbour parasites rather than not. According to the Gates Foundation, which is funding research into vaccines and treatment for such infestations, lymphatic filariasis (one cause of the grossly disfiguring disease commonly known as elephantiasis) affects 120 million people, one-third of whom have serious illness or disability. Eighteen million in Africa and the Americas are infected with onchocerciasis, causing blindness in 270,000 and visual impairment in half a million.

Schistosomiasis, known in one of its forms as bilharzia, infects 200 million people in the developing world. It leads to damage to the bladder and liver, causing renal failure, cancer and cirrhosis. Roundworm infections are more common still: one billion people are believed to be infected with *Ascaris lumbricoides*, a parasite which impairs food digestion and may cause lung disease. A quarter of the entire world's population is believed to be infected with hookworms, which are a common cause of anaemia.

There are other parasites too: strongyloides, trichuria, trichinella, pork and beef tapeworms, and hydatid are all very common indeed, and each has its range of symptoms, from simple lassitude to fits and death. Indeed, tapeworms from pork and beef migrating to the brain are the commonest cause of epilepsy in some parts of the world. The burden of such infections is more clearly demonstrated by a study performed in one African nation, which demonstrated that a single dose in childhood of a drug that kills many intestinal parasites, called levamisole, results in a 10 per cent increase in height and a 5 per cent increase in eventual IQ. Thus parasites make us what we are, and at the same time hinder us from being what we might be.

The intimacy of our connection with these infections has had further consequences for our well-being. The hygiene hypothesis is discussed more fully in Chapter 7. However, it is worth summarising it here during our discussion of parasites. Put briefly, our long evolution with parasites has resulted in the development of a branch of our immune system that controls and suppresses them. Should our lives become too clean, and exclude these organisms, then we risk accidentally triggering the release of undirected and potentially dangerous chemicals which cause the symptoms of allergies like asthma, hayfever and urticaria.

An analogy might be made with traditional building materials. I live in a part of England where many of the houses, including my own, are built of an ancient substance called cob. In essence it is made up of mud, cow dung and straw. Some of these buildings are many hundreds of years old. Provided sympathetic and traditional methods are used to maintain and paint them, so that the cob can 'breathe' and water can expire naturally, they can last indefinitely. However, many have been renovated and painted with clean, modern, waterproof materials. The result is that the cob rots, and in one case at least the house falls down, as happened to a cottage not half a mile from my home. The buildings evolved with the people and the land; our modernity destroys them. So it is with parasites and allergy. Our modern obsession with being clean has caused our immunity to redirect itself at us, sometimes with fatal consequences.

As we shall see in Chapter 7, the ingenuity of humans may be able to direct and correct this imbalance by using harmless extracts of the natural world to set us on the right path again.

Nevertheless the hypothesis confirms the essential theme of this book; we are infectious diseases and we ignore that fact at our peril. We are epidemics of parasites because our genetic make-up and destiny are governed by them. Where we can live is partly defined by them. The huge mortality of malaria defines the demographics of nations. Constant exposure to them restrains our ultimate potential, and we are so used to living alongside them that without their constant challenge our immunity goes haywire in the form of allergy.

These parasitic illnesses are often transmitted by insects. Thus it makes sense for us to move on to consider them next, the charismatic megafauna of the world of infectious diseases.

CHAPTER 4

INSECTS

Eleanor's story

The consequences of contact between humans and insects can be almost viscerally unpleasant. Eleanor was 19 and had recently returned from her gap year before going to university. She had spent her time in Africa, working for a relief organisation. We were called to see her in the accident and emergency department by a rather excited and puzzled surgical colleague. Eleanor had developed a lump over her buttock during the previous week, and had attended to have it examined. She thought it was a developing abscess. Indeed, there was a reddened lump which was oozing clear fluid. The surgeon who was called to see her was on the verge of draining the abscess when he noticed something rather odd about it – something was moving about inside. A fine black thread was protruding from the head of the abscess. When he gently probed it, it abruptly retracted into the pustule.

This was our encounter with the larva of the Tumbu fly. The fine black line was the site of its breathing apparatus, called the spiracle. The female fly of one species, often *Cordylobia anthropophaga*, lays its eggs on sandy ground or clothing. The eggs may not be visible. Almost certainly Eleanor's underwear had become contaminated while she was doing her laundry and hanging her underpants out to dry. The larva, when hatched, then burrows into the skin and after a series of moults drops to the ground where it forms a pupa, hatching as an adult fly after 10–20 days.

We had to be cautious about removing the larva. If they are dragged out too roughly they may rupture and cause an intense and painful inflammatory reaction. The clever trick is to partly suffocate them, to force them to emerge. We smeared a film of liquid paraffin over the spiracle. The gasping larva then began to wriggle from its lair, and we were able to squeeze it gently from its temporary home, intact.

Eleanor made a complete recovery, physically at least. Most people who have suffered a visit from a Tumbu fly struggle to forget the experience. I must admit to some morbid pleasure in passing the larva around to the other nurses and doctors in the department, with an explanation of where it came from and how we had extracted it. The demonstration certainly enlivened the department for that afternoon.

Compared with other larvae, Tumbu are relatively benign. Others of the *Calliphora* family can lay their eggs in the nose. The larvae then migrate through the poor host's tissue, from the nose into the brain and cause death.

The charismatic insect

Insects and their larvae are the charismatic megafauna of the world of infectious diseases. The fascination with the illnesses caused by burrowing larvae is probably out of proportion to their importance as causes of disease. Humans are very often not the main hosts for these infections, and are only coincidentally infected. Tumbu fly, for example, is predominantly a disease of dogs and rodents. It is hardly surprising, though, that humankind should occasionally encounter insects as causes of disease. In some senses, this is not the Era of the Human, or even the Mammal, but the Era of the Insect (although it is even more convincingly the Era of the Microbe).

Of all the world's species that have so far been identified and named, 85 per cent are insects. About 2,000–3,000 new insects are characterised each year, and extrapolating the figures there would appear to be in the order of 20–30 million species, only about 920,000 of which have yet been named. Compare this with our order, the mammals, of which fewer than 4,000 species have been described. The sheer numbers and biomass of insects throughout the world dwarf humanity. In a numerical and quantitative sense, we live on the insects' planet, not they on ours.

Kenneth's story

I was reminded of this statement, one that was impressed upon me while I studied zoology during my early years as a medical student, when I met Kenneth. Here was a man who had a profound sense of kinship with the natural world. He was in his early 40s when I met him. I knew that he would far have preferred to treat his infection with the wide array of crystals, magnets, herbs, tribal nostrums, relaxation techniques and traditional remedies that made up his universe. In fact he had tried many of them before consulting us about his illness, which had begun some weeks previously. His initial problem had been a spreading rash on his thigh. He had treated it himself, and after about three weeks it had vanished. The feeling of tiredness, of lethargy, and of muscle aches that came and went had persisted, however, and it was their occasional association with fever that had triggered his family doctor into sending him to us.

So much of the diagnosis of infectious diseases depends on careful questioning. Kenneth had forgotten about the rash until we asked him directly. He would probably not have mentioned his tendency to sleep outdoors during the summer months, often in woodland, unless we had pursued the question. He liked to commune with the natural world, and to offer his personal apologies to the spirits who he believed inhabited that world in the form of plants and animals. He was apologising for the thoughtless manner in which humans exploit and damage the natural environment; the environment returned the compliment by infecting him with a dangerous and unpleasant bacterium, through the agency of a biting insect.

Kenneth's infection rarely kills, but causes long-term debilitating disease if it is not treated. Its mode of transmission is nauseating to some. On this occasion the warning signals about this apparently new disease – one that is achieving epidemic proportions – were raised by concerned parents.

Worried mothers in Lyme

In 1977 a pair of worried mothers in a semi-rural area of Connecticut drew their local doctor's attention to the large number of cases of arthritis among local children. A team from Yale, led by a rheumatology physician called Allen Steere, was called in to look at the figures. Sure enough the figures did suggest an outbreak: the infection rate among children in this area was 12.2 in 1,000. The symptoms were similar to juvenile rheumatoid arthritis, but this was 100 times the expected prevalence of the disease. There was a further peculiarity. Half of the affected children lived on two roads, which were next to one another, in a densely forested area on the edge of town. Some families were affected more than others. The illness seemed to come on in the summer or early autumn.

When the doctors actively looked for cases – they uncovered 39 – the clusters near dense woodland were exactly matched in a similar community nearby. The evidence pointed to something unpleasant lurking in the woods. The Connecticut town where the two mothers lived was called Old Lyme, and the name of the town was given to the disease, Lyme arthritis. Although there was speculation that the illness was spread by some sort of insect, no cause was identified.

Cut to the early 1980s. Willy Burgdorfer is a Swiss-born entomologist, still living and active in the world of medicine. He was then working at the National Institutes of Health in Hamilton, Montana. His particular interest was Rocky Mountain spotted fever, a disease rather like typhus that is spread by ticks. Burgdorfer and his colleagues Jorge Benach and Edward Bosler had a dangerous task – collecting insects and examining them for diseases that can affect humans. In the autumn of 1981, the team found something new. In the body fluid of two ticks Burgdorfer examined, he identified some slow-moving corkscrew-shaped bacteria.

Burgdorfer looked to his older textbooks. These ticks had been recorded as causing illness before. In Europe it had previously been known as Bannwarth syndrome. His new bacterium – which belonged to the spirochetes, a group of organisms that includes those causing syphilis and Weil's disease – was named *Borrelia burgdorferi* in his honour; Burgdorfer and his colleagues were soon able to prove that it was the cause of the Lyme arthritis.

It soon also became clear that 'arthritis' was not the only manifestation of the illness, nor was it confined to Connecticut or even America. It has been found in 47 of the United States, in Europe, Scandinavia, China, Japan and Australia. Burgdorfer's research showed that records of Lyme-type disease dated back to 1883 in Breslau, Germany, where a physician named Alfred Buchwald described a tick-bite-related skin disorder. In 1909 a physician called Arvid Afzelius described an expanding, ring-like skin rash to the Swedish Society of Dermatology, which he believed had followed the bite of an *Ixodes* tick. There turned out to be a rich vein of literature suggesting a link between tick bites and various illnesses. Disease of the joints had been noted in 1921, neurological problems in 1922, and psychiatric symptoms in 1934. These are all now known to be typical of Lyme.

Getting cross about ticks

Ticks are widespread throughout the world. If you own a dog you may be familiar with them, and have had to extract their bloated, blood-engorged forms from the skin of your pet. Ticks can transmit a variety of illnesses, including an unpleasant paralysis and the exotically named Crimea-Congo haemorrhagic fever. They do so because they feed on the blood of animals. As they feed they regurgitate their stomach contents into their bite. In this fluid there may be a variety of bacteria and viruses. Hard-bodied ticks of the species *Ixodes* are more common in Europe and North America, and it is these that spread Lyme disease.

The insects are tiny before they feed. They lurk on blades of grass or other vegetation, and latch on to passing warm-blooded animals. These may be mice, deer, dogs or birds. The spirochete Burgdorfer saw under his microscope has been found in mosquitoes and deer flies, but as far as is known only the ticks spread the illness to people. It has been claimed that the tick needs to be attached to a person for 24 hours in order to transmit its bacteria (although this is disputed by some). Sometimes a history of tick exposure can be hard to confirm. There are no ticks that feed exclusively on humans.

Although this infection is transmitted by insects, it differs from diseases like Mary's in that it is not the insect itself that does the damage. It is entirely possible to be bitten by a tick and to suffer no consequences at all, or just irritation and a scar. I have included Kenneth's story because his response to his illness reflects something profound about the interaction between man and insect. We have discussed other diseases in the same context – yellow fever, for instance, and sleeping sickness. It is the restless nature of humans to explore and exploit new environments that brings them into contact with unknown (or once known and since almost forgotten) diseases.

In Lyme disease, then, we see classical features of the 'new' epidemics. The encroachment of humans into new habitats, or the alteration of the environment to our own ends, exposes us to exotic, apparently novel infections. Moreover it is sometimes humanity's own actions that provide the precise circumstances that permit the infection to transmit. The persistence of Lyme-infected ticks that may infect humans in many environments relies on the presence of introduced, non-indigenous species. Pheasants, native to Asia, are common hosts to ticks, as are many introduced deer species. If these species had not been imported deliberately, as prey for hunting and shooting, for agriculture or for ornament, tick distribution and the chances of human infection would be very different.

The Lyme bacterium reproduces principally in rodents. While it is of course entirely possible for humans to contract ticks from rodents at grass level, the chances of their being infected are much greater if the tick is brought to a higher level of vegetation by larger animals.

The crucial importance of insects lies in their capacity to act as efficient vectors in numerous epidemic diseases. Malaria, yellow fever, Dengue, typhus, sleeping sickness and relapsing fever are other examples. It is often said that the malarial mosquito is the most dangerous animal on the planet. There are other insects that are capable of causing illness in their own right.

Tumbu is unpleasant and can be intensely itchy and painful, but it rarely kills or causes serious illness. Such is not the case with all of the flies that reproduce through burrowing larvae.

The good insect

Not every invasion by the larvae of insects is to our disadvantage. Some years before starting at medical school I worked as a riding instructor. My duties included grooming the horses of owners who kept their animals in our yard. I recall a fine grey gelding called Pawley, who belonged to a local surgeon. Pawley developed a nasty sore over his withers, the small mound of tissue at the base of the neck. It arose from a badly fitting saddle. The resulting wound became extensive and infected, and the vet struggled to treat it with various antibiotics and creams. We began to worry that Pawley might need an operation. In horses this is not a minor matter: anaesthetising such large animals is a specialist matter requiring expensive facilities.

As we were debating the best way forward Pawley's owner arrived with a small perforated box. He carefully taped it, inverted, over the infected area. Within a few days the wound began to improve, and after a few weeks we were able to remove all the dressings to let the remaining healthy tissue heal. The box had contained maggots. They had eaten all the dead and damaged tissue, including the infecting bacteria, and left healthy tissue behind. Pawley was up and working again after a few short months, albeit with a brand-new expensive fitted saddle.

It has been known for centuries that maggots can assist in the cleaning and healing of infected wounds. Maggot debridement therapy (MDT) first entered modern medical literature in 1931, when the pioneering work of the orthopaedic surgeon William Baer, at Johns Hopkins University in Baltimore, Maryland, was published after his death. It was popular until the mid-1940s, when the miraculous new antibiotics and improved surgical techniques developed in the Second World War appeared to render it obsolete. It was used sporadically in the latter part of the 20th century, but now interest in it is increasing again, principally using the larvae of the green blowfly, *Phaenicia sericata*.

The chief difference between the larvae of blowfly and the larvae of insets that cause disease in humans is that the former fortunately eat only dead tissue. Thus they are ideal for removing dead and decaying tissue from wounds. Leeches may serve a similar function, particularly where the tissues are swollen and blood drainage is restricted by the pressure of the swelling. This is particularly useful in smaller areas like hands, and leeches secrete useful compounds into wounds that break down clots and allow them to be carried away. Indeed, the compound, hirudin, has been purified and is now synthetically made to treat blood clots.

Pressing insects and their larvae into medical service – so called biotherapy – is not confined to maggots. We know from Hindu writings dating from as early as 1000 BC that ants were once pressed into service for closing incisions and small perforations in the intestines, as well as stitching extensive wounds. For instance, species such as the carpenter ant have exceptionally strong jaws. They can be held against the margins of a wound until they have grasped them and drawn the edges together, at which point they are rather ungenerously beheaded. Beetles have been used for the same function. Although of course they are not insects, some fish species that inhabit 'holy ponds' in India are used to treat scabies infections, as well as abscesses and psoriasis.

Insects and their larvae are precisely like the microbes of the world we inhabit in their relationship with us and disease. The vast majority of both numbers and species do us no harm at all, and are indeed vital for the ecology of the planet. They act as prey for larger animals, and as scavengers and recyclers of dead tissue. A tiny number cause disease, either by burrowing into us or by transmitting parasites, viruses and bacteria, but even so, we could not exist without the insects. They pollinate, recycle waste, form prey for our own foods, and some we even eat ourselves. This is a property we shall also encounter in our next group of organisms, the fungi and yeasts.

CHAPTER 5

EPIDEMIC FUNGI
AND YEASTS

Fungi and yeasts are the cause of one of the commonest sexually transmitted infections (STIs) in the world. Many people – including doctors – are surprised by this. If we think of fungi at all in a medical context, we think of hallucinogenic magic mushrooms, poisonous toadstools, and perhaps 'black building' syndrome (the condition where people believe their health is affected by moulds in buildings). Most doctors are familiar with them causing infections in patients undergoing chemotherapy for cancers, or those who have damaged immunity for some other reason. These types of infection are rare by epidemic standards, but they can be very nasty and are frequently fatal. But the most frequently encountered fungal infection is a rather different one. It has undoubtedly reached epidemic proportions, and it can cause pain, embarrassment and even terror.

Lucy's story

Lucy was 16. Like many of her schoolfriends she was beginning to experiment with sex. In fact by the standards of the time hers was a relatively late adventure. The majority of British and western young people begin to embark on sexual intercourse at a younger age than this: 13 is the average age in many areas. Lucy was a shy girl, and took some time to approach her local genito-urinary (GU) medicine clinic with her problem, of which she was deeply ashamed. She had developed sore, painful and reddened areas around her genitals. She was convinced that she had acquired gonorrhoea, herpes or chlamydia, the infections that she had learnt about in her lessons about sex in school. Naturally she was also petrified that she might have acquired HIV.

GU medicine clinics have advanced considerably in recent years. When I was a medical student there used to be a bench in an open corridor on which patients waiting for their appointments would sit, under a large sign saying 'Sexually Transmitted Infection Clinic'. I wonder how many anxious sufferers were deterred by the bench of shame. Nowadays most clinics make some effort to allow patients some discretion. As a consequence of changing sexual standards these clinics are often hopelessly swamped, but they are generally less off-putting than they used to be. Even so, Lucy did not find it easy to make her way to the department and explain her problem. Her terror was evident in her stammering and tearfulness.

One of the pleasures of working in these clinics is the possibility of instant diagnosis and thus instant reassurance. STIs can have characteristic physical symptoms and appearances on examination, and simple swabs examined under the microscope can reveal the cause of a problem right there and then. There was no real difficulty with Lucy: her reddened and sore-looking genitals were typical. A careful inspection of some tissue smeared on a glass slide and stained with one of the oldest techniques – the Gram stain – revealed characteristic dark, almost black organisms with unmistakable features. We could tell instantly that these were not bacteria. When bacteria divide and reproduce, their offspring are an identical size to their parents. The microbes we were looking at divided with a daughter cell that was considerably smaller. Some of them had elongated, leggy protuberances quite unlike bacteria; there were also tell-tale spores present. We had no difficulty in identifying this as vulvo-vaginal candida, more commonly known as thrush.

Lucy was hugely relieved. Thrush is a very common infection, easily treated. Naturally we took care to ensure that she had a clean bill of health from the other sexually acquired infections, and she left the clinic with a prescription for some anti-fungals and a spring in her step. Medicine is not always about curing serious illness: sometimes reassuring the worried well and treating minor illnesses is just as gratifying.

The shameful fungus

GU medicine and sexual health clinics tend to skirt around the notion of candida as a sexually transmitted disease, for obvious reasons. The stigma associated with an STI is potent, and can cause untold damage to self-esteem and to personal human relationships. There is no doubt that candida can be transmitted between sexual partners; males and females may both have symptomatic infection, and often both partners require treatment to eradicate the yeast. I can tell you, though, that were we to tell our patients in such clinics that they had an STI, chaos would ensue.

I once delivered a lecture to a group of family doctors entitled 'Common Infectious Diseases'. There was near-mutiny in the ranks when I stated that candida was the world's most common sexually acquired infection. 'Candida's not an STI!' they chorused. Most think of it as being introduced from the patient's own mouth or intestine, and taking over a new area as a consequence of disruption of the local organisms which should live there. Still others believe that the world's most common STI is caused by the parasite *Trichomonas vaginalis* or by the virus *Herpes simplex*. But by almost any definition – an organism that can cause pain and distress, and that can pass between people during intercourse – candida can be a sexually transmitted disease. And it is very, very common. Significantly for Lucy, the contraceptive pill can make women vulnerable to it.

What candidiasis really reflects is something else about our immersion in, and intimate association with, the microbes that surround and cover us. In the normal state, there are bacteria inhabiting the interior of the female genitals in huge numbers. These are the lactobacilli. They prefer the acid environment of the vaginal vault, and they contribute to that acidity by turning glucose into lactic acid. About half of the acidity is provided by the bacteria, the other half by the person. The production of those acids is sensitive to hormones such as oestrogen, hence the effect of Lucy's contraceptive pill. This acidity makes the environment hostile to other bacteria and fungi; it provides some protection against STIs like chlamydia and gonorrhoea, and invasion by less healthy organisms like candida and others.

Lactobacilli are also capable of producing agents that are toxic to other organisms. When the normal physiology is disrupted these lactobacilli recede and a 'vacant ecological niche' is created, which can be invaded more easily. This is a phenomenon that also occurs elsewhere in the human body – on the skin, for example, and in our intestines. In terms of numbers, bacteria are more likely to protect us from disease than cause it.

At first sight this seems straightforward enough. So-called probiotics protect us from disease; harmless bacteria form a colonising army of friendly forces that deter more dangerous disease-causing organisms. However, this is only a half of the story. Lactobacilli are perfectly capable of causing disease. Should they spill over into a 'sterile' site like the brain they may be as dangerous as many other bacteria. But they are tolerated, even encouraged, in some sites like the vagina and intestine. This means that they have been inspected by the cells of immunity and permitted to remain. Inevitably this is not a one-off inspection; the bacteria will reproduce and present a constant challenge to immunity.

In a sense the recognition of these bacteria, as distinct from fungi, represents a kind of immune tolerance identical to the way we recognise our own cells as 'self', as being us. If we recognise certain bacteria as being self, and the loss of those bacteria encourages a state of fungal disease, what is the difference between them and us? As we saw in the section on bacteria, the ability of bacteria to persist unchallenged is an even more active process, where they signal to us via hormones to let them be. Candida do not do so; that is why their presence leads to inflammation.

The elusive candida syndrome

While we are addressing candida and epidemics, we should consider for a moment the so-called 'candida syndrome' which has received much press coverage in recent years. Put simply, candida syndrome is said to be excessive colonisation of the gut with yeasts like candida. It has been held to be responsible for an enormous variety of problems. One website I found attributed over 90 possible symptoms to candida syndrome, ranging from headaches to hypothyroidism to lupus (a potentially serious, even fatal, condition where the body attacks itself, one of the so-called auto-immune diseases). Included in this list is the unintentionally comical assertion that 'symptoms may be worse after waking'. Apart from nightmares, is there one that isn't?

Given the huge variety of possible manifestations of the syndrome, it is not surprising that one practitioner claims that 'The incidence of yeast syndrome is remarkably high. In my practice signs and symptoms suggesting yeast syndrome are present in 1/2 of new patients.' He also goes on to say:

Candida syndrome is still unaccepted by some medical doctors. The habit of the medical establishment, in general, is to not accept as real any symptom complex which they do not under-stand. The effects of chronic yeast infestation in the intestine are so widespread in the body that it does not at first seem logical that one thing could cause all this. Many a patient have been branded hypochondriac, malingering, neurotic, and hysteric who appeared in doctors' offices with this complex, confusing symptomatology. One of the symptoms is irritability and this quality has tended to alienate doctors, leaving both doctor and patient frustrated. Also, doctors are accustomed to think that if routine blood tests show nothing, then nothing is wrong. Chronic yeast, in fact, shows nothing on routine blood tests.

What should we make of an epidemic of a condition, supposedly caused by yeasts, that affects half of all one doctor's patients yet can produce just about any symptom, ranging from hypothyroidism to an itchy rectum? When I read the extensive list of possible manifestations of the syndrome, a small, gullible part of me was thinking, 'I have many of these symptoms. Maybe I have candida syndrome.' Fortunately I have been able to pull myself back from the brink – but why? What makes me so certain that candida syndrome is bunkum?

There is no question that one of the greatest achievements of the 20th century was the conquest, however temporary, of diseases of infection. In the 19th century probably a third of all deaths were due to infections of one sort or another. Chief among these was tuberculosis. I mention this bacterial disease because the discoverer of the tubercle bacillus – Robert Koch – is crucial to modern understanding of whether or not a particular organism is responsible for a particular disease. Armed with this knowledge, you can decide for yourself whether candida syndrome is correctly attributed.

Koch realised that to tackle diseases of infection it would be crucial to prove beyond doubt that you were attacking the correct target. To this end in 1884 he and Frederic Loeffler devised a series of rules which had to be satisfied before you could make the claim with certainty. These are known as 'Koch's postulates', and, in slightly modified form, they survive to this day. They are:

1 The organism must be found in all animals suffering from the disease, but not in healthy animals.
2 The organism must be isolated from a diseased animal and grown in pure culture.
3 The cultured organism should cause disease when introduced into a healthy animal.
4 The organism must be reisolated from the experimentally infected animal.

Koch originally applied the postulates to tuberculosis and anthrax, but acknowledged during his own lifetime that the second part of rule 1 might not universally apply. He realised that healthy animals (and humans) may be carriers of disease. We have encountered this rather dramatically in the story of Typhoid Mary, where an apparently healthy woman infected a number of people with a lethal bacterium. Subsequently researchers have demonstrated many examples of diseases that they are certain are caused by an agent which turns out not to be amenable to culture. Hepatitis C is a good example, as is syphilis. Neither can be grown in the laboratory (at the time of writing). Thus it may not be necessary to fulfil all the rules.

Consider now the case for candida syndrome. Superficially it might seem that it fulfils all the criteria except number 3. Ironically, candida would fail the part of rule 1 that Koch himself abandoned, because candida is found in the intestines of all healthy humans. Candida will therefore satisfy rule 2, and definitely be found in the intestines of every animal (human) suffering from the disease. We can isolate candida in pure culture from that same source and thus satisfy the second part of rule 2. We can definitely satisfy rule 4, and reisolate candida from an experimentally infected human, because every human has candida in his or her intestine.

Now let us suppose we choose some other quality of sufferers from candida syndrome. For the sake of argument, let it be the presence of a detectable heartbeat. Let us try to predict from our two tests which patient has candida syndrome compared with a group of controls. The answer is that neither quality will have any predictive value. Because everybody has a heartbeat and everybody has candida in their intestines, neither will help us.

Of course we would never have expected the presence of a detectable heartbeat to help us in our identification of patients with candida syndrome, because there simply can be no logical connection between the two. At some level, then, we must expect our possible disease-causing organism to follow some basic principle of cause and effect. Beyond a vague mention of 'toxic substances' produced by candida there is no such causative association. Candida is a relatively non-toxic organism. It causes disease only when present in the wrong site (the intestine being the right one) or where the immunity is grossly damaged. As a general rule, the human body tolerates toxic organisms poorly. It is the function of the immune response to expel them.

Supporters of the candida syndrome as a diagnosis sometimes cite excessive colonisation of the intestine by candida. In that case it would be very straightforward to quantify. Counting numbers and types of organisms in faeces is not difficult, although it is certainly unpleasant. There is no such evidence. Some advocates of the syndrome also claim that there is a more complex imbalance present, with other 'anaerobic bacteria' (also present in every intestine) being responsible, as well as mercury in dental fillings. The problem with all of this is that is impossible to disprove. I understand that this is not a view that will be popular everywhere, but I shall stick my neck out. There is no conclusive proof of the existence of a candida syndrome, and for the reasons I have explained, there almost certainly never will be.

Black buildings and weary humans

Nor is candida syndrome the only fungal infection that is believed to cause such vague epidemics. Nigel – a librarian – came to see us because he felt tired all the time. This is a common referral to an infectious diseases department. Some such departments accept patients with a possible diagnosis of ME, or chronic fatigue syndrome. One theory claims that the syndrome is an abnormal response to infection, probably a virus.

During our prolonged conversation Nigel voiced his anxieties about his living accommodation. Librarians are not well paid. London is an expensive city. He was concerned that his symptoms had been caused by a toxic-looking mould that had started to creep around the cupboard under the stairs of his dingy bed-sitting room. Nigel thought he might be suffering the effects of black building syndrome, a diagnosis which has reached apparently epidemic proportions in some quarters.

Sometimes the medical profession comes head to head with vigorously held public opinion on such matters. There is no doubt that moulds and fungi can cause human disease, as I have demonstrated above. Moulds are common and important causes of allergic problems. About 5 per cent of individuals are believed to have some allergic airway symptoms from moulds over their lifetime. However, it should be remembered that moulds are not the commonest causes of these symptoms, and further that outdoor moulds, rather than indoor ones, are the most important. For almost all allergic individuals, the reactions will be limited to inflammation of the nasal passages or asthma; sinusitis may occur secondarily as a result of obstruction. Fatigue and headaches are not part of these symptoms.

Fungi may cause other diseases among humans. Superficial fungal infections of the skin and nails are relatively common, but those infections are easily treated and generally get better without problems. Fungal infections of parts of the body deeper than the skin are rare, and in general are limited to persons with severely impaired immune systems. The leading pathogenic fungi for persons with healthy immune function are called *Blastomyces, Coccidioides, Cryptococcus* and *Histoplasma*. We shall discuss them later. They may be encountered indoors when they are carried there by the inward flow of outdoor air, but normally they do not grow there.

The cause of black building syndrome is believed to be those moulds that propagate indoors. There is no doubt that these moulds may under some conditions produce substances called mycotoxins, which can adversely affect living cells and organisms by a variety of mechanisms. Mycotoxins are known to be toxic; there is even some evidence that they have been used as bioweapons in, for instance, the Vietnam War. Occupational diseases are also recognised in association with inhalation exposure to fungi, bacteria and other organic matter, usually in industrial or agricultural settings.

There are plenty of publications that seek to draw a link between certain moulds – and one in particular, *Stachybotrys chartarum* – and certain disease states. That link remains weak and unproven, particularly when mycotoxins are included in the chain. *S. chartarum* may produce mycotoxins under appropriate growth conditions. Nevertheless, years of intensive study have failed to demonstrate that exposure to it in home, school or office environments is a cause of adverse human health effects. It has been investigated by measuring people's exposure in the indoor environment, by exposure of animals, and by dose-rate calculation. All suggest that it is highly unlikely that anyone could ever inhale a toxic dose of mycotoxins in an indoor environment, even if they were among the most vulnerable.

Mould spores are present in all indoor environments and cannot be eliminated from them. Moulds can easily grow on normal building materials and furnishings. The association with disease is almost certainly related to their unsightly appearance and the smells they may release. As we have said, some moulds may sensitise and produce allergic responses in allergic individuals. However, except for people with severely impaired immune systems, indoor mould is not a source of fungal infections. Current scientific evidence simply does not support the proposition that human health has been adversely affected by inhaled naturally occurring mycotoxins.

Other fungi are more capable of causing disease in huge numbers; the agents of conditions such as athlete's foot are enormously common. Cuts in the skin can lead to secondary infection with more dangerous bacteria, but generally these are an annoyance rather than a dangerous infection. There are fungi that are responsible for catastrophic epidemics among animals. *Batrachochytrium dendrobatidis* is a fungal disease responsible for the death and extinction of millions of frogs and other reptiles, believed to be accelerated by global warming. However, this book is primarily concerned with human disease, and this will not be considered further. As for Nigel – he turned out to have an underactive thyroid.

Juan's story

The experience of humans and serious fungal infections is more closely reflected by the story of Juan. He was a young man in his 20s who had travelled around his native Bolivia on a motorcycle. About a year before we encountered him he had come off his bike and grazed his elbow. At the site of the wound he had developed livid purple blotches and raised bumps. He had been consulting a dermatologist in Bolivia, but by the time we were called to see him he was in need of more than a skin specialist. He was admitted to our intensive care unit with persistent epileptic seizures and variable consciousness. The scans of his brain revealed large areas of abnormal tissue in his brain. His chest X-ray also showed patches of shadowing, which suggested that something had infiltrated his lungs.

Juan deteriorated rapidly. We urgently asked our pathology department to explore the nature of the lesions on his skin. We had to seek confirmation from a pathologist who specialised in infectious diseases before we could be certain: Juan had a very rare fungal disease called coccidioidomycosis. Sadly, his disease was too far advanced for us to cure him, and he died within a week of appearing in our hospital. He had driven the spores of the fungus into his arm during his fall on that road in Bolivia. The organism had slowly multiplied there. While it was causing him enough discomfort to consult a dermatologist, it was also insidiously sending off tiny satellites to his lungs and brain.

The key to the difference between fungi and other infectious agents is contained in Juan's story. In essence, with a few rare exceptions, fungi do not readily transmit from person to person as viruses and bacteria may. This is why they generally do not cause epidemics. Laboratories do need to be cautious when examining and culturing tissue that is suspected of harbouring coccidioidomycosis or histoplasmosis, but generally the diseases are contracted by direct contact with the agent in the environment. With the exceptions of candidiasis and childhood ringworm these are organisms that thrive in the world and only cause illness in humans almost by accident.

Nevertheless the incidence of serious fungal disease is increasing, and has been for some decades. The next story illustrates why this is so.

Ahmed's story

Ahmed was 62. He had been a diabetic since the age of 11, and needed to use insulin to control his condition. He had recently been suffering headaches and pain in the face, with occasional fevers. He had also noticed a swelling at the back of his mouth, on the palate. When his family doctor saw it, he found it so alarming that he arranged for Ahmed to be seen urgently by ear, nose and throat specialists.

Ahmed had a large black-looking ulcer at the back of his throat, and some of the tissues seemed to have disappeared. The specialists called us as soon as they had the pathologist's report on the tissue that they had removed. Under the microscope they had seen the typical branching growths of a condition called rhinocerebral mucormycosis. If it is left unchecked it can erode right through the skull bones into the brain, causing death.

We immediately started to treat Ahmed with anti-fungal agents, and asked the surgeons to remove as much tissue as possible. To cure this fungal infection the tissue has to be stripped back right to the bone and sometimes beyond. Because of Ahmed's diabetes his kidneys were in poor shape, and we had to use the most expensive antifungal agent in the formulary to protect them from further damage, because the standard, cheaper antifungal agent can be toxic to the kidneys. It took many months to cure him, and eventually he left hospital with a metal plate called an obturator to cover the gaping hole in his palate. We calculated as he left that his cure had cost roughly the equivalent of his weight in gold.

Attacking the weakened

The key to the modern epidemic of fungal disease lies in the very first sentence of Ahmed's story. There is an increased number of people now alive who have severely damaged immunity. At one extreme this includes patients with cancer, whose bone marrow has been deliberately destroyed in the hope of eradicating the disease. This leaves them open to many infections with feebly pathogenic organisms that the healthy would shrug off. At the less severe end of the spectrum are for example people with diabetes, who are also more at risk from all sorts of infections, including serious fungal diseases.

We should remember that diabetes has only recently become a treatable condition. Until the discovery of insulin in 1921 by Banting and Best, the insulin-dependent variety at least was uniformly fatal. Many people with HIV/AIDS, serious burns and trauma victims, premature babies, the very young and the very old would also not be alive were it not for modern medicine. Collected together they form a sizeable group of people, and this explains the steady increase in the number of fungal infections encountered every year.

This epidemic is therefore human-made, but it is one in which we may feel a perverse sense of pride. Ironically fungi have caused an epidemic among this new group, the people who might otherwise have died, because they are simply not very good at causing disease. They do not cause disease in the otherwise healthy, because they lack the claws, teeth and muscle of their more pathogenic cousins in the world of bacteria and viruses. In this respect fungi are exceptions to the theme of this book. Broadly fungi have not evolved as human or animal pathogens, with the exception of a few generally fairly harmless skin organisms such as the ones that cause athlete's foot.

The existence of large numbers of immune-compromised people is recent, and irrelevant in evolutionary terms. Should we lose the ability to keep people with such gaps in immunity alive, then this is an epidemic that would vanish. The rest of us could quite happily live among the vast majority of fungi without suffering any ill-effects. It is only when the immune system is damaged and disrupted that they can slip into our bodies and make us ill.

The witch fungus

Elizabeth was nine years old when her symptoms began; they were identical to those of her cousin Abigail. Their illness came on during a cold January. The symptoms of the disease were peculiar feelings under the skin, followed by babbling, meaningless speech, confusion and fits. The rural area where they lived had never encountered anything like this before, and the local physicians were utterly baffled. Ultimately the outbreak affected eight children, but it claimed 25 lives, all adults. None of the adults had the original illness. It was to be a very long time before a compelling hypothesis implicating a fungus was put forward to explain this epidemic, the cause of which has never been conclusively proven. The reasons for this may become clear when the date and location of the episode are revealed. This was Salem, Massachusetts in 1692.

At the time the disorder was famously believed to be a consequence of witchcraft. Elizabeth Parris was the daughter of the local priest. The first to be accused were his slave, Tituba, and two older local women who were considered to be of poor repute. By the time the governor of the colony, Sir William Phipps, called the accusations and executions to an end in September, 150 people had been arrested, 20 had been executed and five had died in custody.

The Salem witch trials were immortalised by Arthur Miller in his play *The Crucible*. One evening in the early 1970s Linnda Caporael, a behavioural psychologist at New York's Rensselaer Polytechnic Institute, saw the play. It triggered a memory: years ago as a child she had read of a similar episode in France. This occurred in 1951 in Pont-Saint-Esprit, a small town on the Rhone with 4,400 inhabitants. That town was gripped by an outbreak of bizarre behaviour among its citizens. Some hallucinated, others hurled themselves from buildings, children attacked their parents, and men ran through the streets convinced they were being pursued by their enemies. Seven died. Could the two episodes share a cause, thought Caporael? She remembered that a cause had been suggested for the French incident. That autumn had been uncommonly rainy and there were perfect conditions for fungus to grow on the wet grain. Analyses done at the time had shown that the fungus *Claviceps purpurea*, the poison ergot, was growing in the area, and the hypothesis was that its toxins had caused the strange behaviour.

There is no doubt that ergotism (the name given to poisoning by *Claviceps purpurea*) can reproduce the symptoms described both at Pont-Saint-Esprit and at Salem. Ergotism was once common, to the extent that it was assigned the name St Anthony's Fire. The cure was said to be pilgrimage to the Alps, where *Claviceps* did not grow. Whether the witches of Salem were under the influence of ergot is another matter. There are plenty who doubt it and advance more psycho-social theories. It would be impossible to prove, and even the diagnosis at Pont-Saint-Esprit has been questioned – some say it was really mercury poisoning. The hallucinogenic drug LSD can be derived from ergot, but this is not quite the same as saying that LSD from ergot was responsible for what happened at Salem, as some have claimed. For our purposes it is enough to say that the toxic products of fungi are capable of causing small epidemics. Ergot poisoning is on the list of possible agents of bioterrorism, and indeed it was used a weapon in antiquity. Nor is ergot the only fungus that is so toxic. *Aspergillus* species are capable of producing substances called aflatoxins which are implicated in cancers.

Toxic products like ergot have much in common with penicillin. Both are substances produced naturally which have therapeutic value. Ergot is – or used to be – used for the treatment of migraines; it is an alkaloid upon which many drugs are based. Moulds produce penicillin to protect their ecological niches from bacteria. Ergot alkaloids have antibacterial action also; whether this is their primary function is not clear, but it is unlikely that the chemical is produced in such quantities without purpose. Very little happens in nature without an evolutionary reason.

The allergy epidemic

In the section on allergies we discuss another method by which fungi cause disease: they can trigger such reactions as asthma. The modern epidemic of asthma and allergy can also be said in part to be human-made, as is explained on pages 180–85, where I discuss the hygiene hypothesis. The capacity of fungal spores to trigger allergy is only indirectly connected to that hypothesis, and such diseases occurred before our modern obsession with cleanliness. The condition of asthma as a consequence of allergy to fungal spores is nevertheless very common indeed. Some authorities claim that 25 per cent of asthma sufferers actually have a reaction to a common fungus called aspergillus, a condition more properly known as allergic bronchopulmonary aspergillosis.

In the other chapters of this book the consistent theme is that humans are infectious diseases. In the context of fungi and yeasts, our exposure to them has been massively to our advantage. Imagine a world without baker's yeast. It has been argued that the development of bread as a prepared, storable foodstuff with ingredients that may be kept for use when convenient was the key moment in the development and expansion of human civilisation. Penicillin, of course, is a product of the *Penicillium* fungus, as are many of the antibiotics on which we have relied. *Penicillium* is capable of causing disease, as is *Saccharomyces* (bakers' and brewers' yeast), but compared with the benefits these organisms have given us, these problems are trivial.

We are what we eat

The rather eccentric headmaster of my secondary school used to carry a plastic bag full of fungi about with him in the autumn. Periodically he would summon a schoolboy at random, then instruct him to eat a piece of foul-looking forest mushroom. He would then observe the child intently for a few moments before nodding and moving on. Of course he knew that these were not lethal toadstools, but he enjoyed the discomfiture of the nervous victims.

Fungi could be described as the cattle of epidemics, compared with the sharks and tigers of some bacteria and viruses. If you swim with sharks or walk among tigers you have a lower chance of getting away with it, depending on how close your contact. Fungi in contrast are generally benign, useful even, but people are occasionally killed by stampeding cows or an enraged bull.

We shall end this chapter on fungi and disease with an intriguing observation about another, unrelated epidemic. I discuss mad cow disease elsewhere (see chapter 8). The agent of that illness, and related diseases like human vCJD (variant Creutzfelt-Jacob Disease, also discussed in chapter 8) and kuru, is the odd man out of the epidemic world, because it contains no genetic material. This is the prion, and as far as we know it is simply a variety of protein that causes disease by triggering distortions in other proteins. For a while it appeared that prions only caused disease in mammals. However, in the late 1990s it became apparent that fungi and plants contain proteins that closely resemble prions. Not only do they contain them, they appear to use them to their own advantage.

There is a species of fungus called *Podospora anserina*. It is capable of forming cooperative colonies, much like the biofilms we encountered in Chapter 2. The process of cooperation involves sharing nutrients; it is in the reproductive interests of the colony to ensure that only similar organisms are allowed to enlist. This other fungus uses prions to regulate the species of fungi that are permitted to join the collective. The prion protein kills off unsuitable candidates by triggering exactly the same distortion in proteins that occurs in diseases like vCJD and mad cow. In other words, fungi appear to have evolved prions to reinforce species selection in the sharing of nutrients. Compare that with the method by which prion disease is believed to have entered the human life cycle – by people eating infected cows who in turn had been fed cattle proteins. Prions may have evolved to prevent the miscegenation of species. Fungi have much to tell us about who we are; if this hypothesis turns out to be correct, then what we are is very like them.

We now move on to the diseases that follow disasters, either human-induced or natural.

CHAPTER 6

THE FOUR HORSEMEN

Gerry's story

Gerry was a middle-aged, middle-class, pleasant, slightly over-weight and bespectacled gentleman I encountered shortly after his return from South Africa, where he had stayed in the farmhouse of an ostrich ranch. He had taken a safari on the trip, and had camped out in the bush. On returning to Britain he began to feel a little unwell, with a fever and headache. He also had a slightly troubling cough. Shortly before he visited our hospital he developed a widespread fine rash over his chest and limbs.

Diagnosis of infectious diseases can sometimes be gratifyingly rapid. The story he told me fitted neatly with my suspicions, and the faint fluffy changes on the chest x-ray supported my provisional assumption. When I examined him carefully I found a tiny black spot above his right buttock; Gerry hadn't noticed it. We had to wait a few days for the confirmatory tests to return from the lab, but my initial hunch was confirmed. Gerry had wandered into the territory of other creatures and paid a small price. The small black mark on his bottom was the site of the tick bite. He was easily cured with antibiotics.

Gerry was lucky in a way, since there are many serious diseases carried by ticks, including Crimea-Congo haemorrhagic fever (also harboured by ostriches), which is untreatable and frequently fatal. Gerry's disease was African tick typhus, which is a close relative of one of the great scourges of war zones and the sites of natural disasters, louse-borne, or epidemic typhus.

One disaster leads to another

We have become depressingly familiar with floods, tsunamis, earthquakes, wars and famines. Barely a year seems to pass without some benighted spot suffering casualties in their tens of thousands. With the possible exception of wars and famines, these are generally not the fault of humans, although of course measures can be taken to reduce the hazards, such as earthquake-proof buildings, tsunami warning systems and drainage schemes. Further, scientists who study climate change patterns warn us that storm patterns are affected by increasing temperatures, and there could be more and worse disasters in the future as a result.

Such issues are beyond the scope of this book. What we shall consider here are the consequences of such disasters, in the form of epidemic infectious diseases. It should become apparent that these are preventable 'natural' disasters. There is no reason that a tsunami or an earthquake should automatically be followed by mass outbreaks of cholera, typhoid or typhus. These result from a failure of public health and of rapid aid provision in the form of shelter and food, and in at least one case from the failure to offer routine, cheap vaccination properly in advance of a disaster.

We should begin by dismissing a myth about dead bodies and epidemics. Humans generally feel a profound, visceral, almost atavistic distaste for the dead bodies of their own species. Many cultures demand rapid disposal of the remains of a deceased person. The popular understanding of the reason for this is that decaying corpses pose a risk to the health of the living. Perhaps surprisingly, this is generally not the case. It should be recalled that three things are required to ensure transmission of infections: a susceptible victim, a route of transmission and the presence of the infecting agent. Generally after natural disasters the cause of death will have been trauma. Unless the victim was coincidentally suffering from an infection, the corpse will not present a risk.

Even for someone handling the cadaver of a person who has died of infectious disease, the risk is small, with the possible exception of some viruses that are highly infectious in blood, like Lassa, Marburg, Ebola and Crimea-Congo haemorrhagic fever. There may be a higher risk in handling large numbers of corpses after a major catastrophe, where there can also be large volumes of spilled blood. The principal diseases that pose such a hazard are hepatitis B virus, hepatitis C virus and HIV. The agents of diarrhoea and mycobacterium tuberculosis are also a potential hazard. Although each of these can be responsible for epidemics, and as a result they are discussed in this book, none (apart from diarrhoea) generally follows a natural disaster.

There is a common view that when corpses float in bodies of water during floods, there is a risk of cholera. This is only the case when the floodwaters previously harboured the cholera bacterium, and those waters contaminate the drinking water supply. I live in an area of Britain prone to flooding; the risk of cholera following a flood, even if people are killed and their bodies float unrecovered for some time, is effectively zero. Floods in Bangladesh (as happened in 1971) have a very different outcome, because cholera lurks in the water there. In a sense this is contrary to the theme of this book: humans are not epidemics when they are dead. There is one possible exception to this rule, but the circumstances that might lead to an epidemic occur only in particular and specific circumstances, and the connection with the human corpse is only tangential.

Iris and the tsunami victims

Iris was 83 when she died. I never met her, but like almost every doctor who worked in our hospital, I knew her story because it was typed out and posted on the noticeboard of the doctors' station in the emergency department as a reminder. She was long dead by the time I read about her. She had sought help for her peculiar and progressive loss of ability to use her limbs. Naturally she was admitted for investigations, and a number of possible rare diagnoses were considered. However, none of them fitted the case, and meanwhile her symptoms progressed rapidly.

A relatively junior doctor stumbled on the diagnosis almost by chance. He happened to ask her husband whether she had had any injury involving soil in the recent past. He answered that she had – she had cut her finger on a rose thorn while pruning. With horror her doctors realised that she had a disease more or less banished from the West, tetanus. Despite the best available treatment, involving artificial ventilation and intensive care, Iris died.

In the aftermath of the Boxing Day tsunami of 2004, many deaths resulted unnecessarily from tetanus. This is a disease which has effectively vanished from the developed nations; a single case in Britain would almost certainly make national newspaper headlines. The condition results from the contamination of a wound by the tetanus bacterium, *Clostridium tetani*. This bacterium may or may not be present in the intestines of humans; however, that is not its main source. *Clostridium tetani* inhabits the soil, usually passed there in animal faeces. Many hapless victims tossed impotently through the surging waters of the tsunami were hit and injured by floating debris, and where this resulted in an open wound – even a tiny one – the conditions were there for some of them to be infected by the tetanus bacillus.

Whether the source of the bacillus was the intestine of flood victims, or far more likely, the soil, contact with those tiny wounds was enough to permit the organism to release its load of deadly paralysing toxin. The mortality from tetanus in Thailand was zero; in that country there is an effective system of health care, and almost everyone is vaccinated against it in childhood. In Indonesia, where healthcare is more rudimentary, hundreds died of the preventable disease, many of them children.

Older people who work with the soil often develop natural, if unreliable, immunity to tetanus. Iris is a sad example of that unreliability: she had been vaccinated but she still died of the disease. Occasional cases like hers occur in the elderly in developed countries, where immunity has waned. Nevertheless this further illustrates my point. Although it is obvious that bodies should be collected and interred or cremated rapidly for aesthetic, cultural, religious and personal reasons, the risk of their transmitting infectious disease is slight.

The huddled starving masses

It is the living who pose more of a hazard. The factors that do permit epidemics to develop after disasters are mostly related to the mass displacement of malnourished survivors, who are often crowded into makeshift camps, in unsanitary conditions, with contaminated water supplies. There are three main sources of epidemics in these circumstances: respiratory diseases, transmitted by droplets of contaminated air that are inhaled; diarrhoeal diseases acquired through contaminated food and water supplies (this includes typhoid fever, which generally does not cause diarrhoea but is acquired by the same route); and diseases spread by biting insects such as mosquitoes, lice, sandflies and ticks.

From a scientific perspective there is more to susceptibility to these diseases than merely being part of a huddled starving mass. The stress of a natural disaster contributes significantly to the susceptibility of an individual to disease. Stress results in excessive production of a hormone, a steroid called cortisol.

This is the opposite variety of steroid to that used by body-builders, and results in the withering of muscle rather than growth. It is a normal physiological response, and is an evolutionary mechanism: in these circumstances people's metabolism changes so that vital organs like the brain, heart and lungs are conserved at the expense of muscle. Cortisol has particular and specific effects on the immunity of our cells. It has long been known that times of war result in an increased incidence of diseases like tuberculosis. We also now know that animals subjected to stress will be more likely to develop infections, and that the course of those infections will be different, usually more severe, when they are in a state of prolonged stress.

The diseases that arise after environmental or civil catastrophes are those that already existed in small numbers among the disrupted community, but which can then spread more rapidly because of the large numbers of stressed people crammed together, those diseases that are present in the environment and to which the survivors are newly exposed, or a combination of both. As a consequence, the prior state of health of the survivors has a major impact on the outcome.

After Hurricane Katrina caused widespread flooding in New Orleans and devastation in surrounding states in August 2005, the main hazard was diarrhoeal and respiratory illness caused by a number of bacteria and viruses which are common in any event. The incidence of such illnesses increased – there were 20 clusters of diarrhoeal disease in refugee centres in Louisiana, and about 1,000 cases in Mississippi and Texas, according to the American Centers for Disease Control. There was a small number of cases of skin infections, some of which were caused by bacteria present in seawater, some by bacteria like MRSA. All known cases of tuberculosis were carefully followed up. There was no increase in cases.

Rich man, poor man

Outbreaks may arise where large numbers of survivors are displaced into areas where mosquito or insect-borne diseases are common. In the United States such outbreaks have occurred, albeit rarely. After the Red River flood which affected Minnesota in 1975 there were 55 cases of western equine encephalitis and 12 of St Louis encephalitis. Both are viral illnesses which can kill, and are spread by mosquitoes. Of the 11 subsequent major floods in the United States that have been surveyed, there was no similar outbreak among humans. There were a number of cases among animals, including horses and emus. Nevertheless the United States broadly avoided mass outbreaks of disease following natural disaster in the 20th century.

Let us contrast this state of affairs with disasters in countries where the previous health of the population was less good, and where poverty and poor infrastructure meant that the relief effort was less well coordinated. In November 1998 Hurricane Mitch struck Central America. During the period from 29 October to 3 November, the hurricane dropped colossal amounts of rainfall in Honduras and Nicaragua, with some claiming that up to 75 inches fell. Nearly 11,000 people were killed and over 8,000 were left unaccounted for. In Guatemala in the months prior to the hurricane there had been an outbreak of cholera. Between January and October in the pre-hurricane period, 2,530 cases were reported. The weekly average was 59. During November a total of 1,941 cases were reported, a weekly average of 485. By 2 December, the Ministry of Public Health reported a total of 38 outbreaks and 33 deaths as a result of cholera. The source of infection in almost all outbreaks was contaminated food.

Similar outbreaks, although less marked, occurred in El Salvador, Belize, Honduras and Nicaragua. That last nation also endured an outbreak of Weil's disease, or leptospirosis, an unpleasant bacterial disease spread from the urine of rats. Following Hurricane Frederick in 1979 similar outbreaks of cholera, typhoid and malaria occurred in the Dominican Republic.

Man's inhumanity and disease

I have yet to encounter a patient with cholera. In its most aggressive form it results in a most distressing condition where diarrhoea is profuse and so dilute as to resemble rice-water. Death is by dehydration. As can be seen from the above figures, death is not universal. However, it is both a preventable and nowadays a curable condition; indeed, it was the first disease to be controlled by what we now understand by public health. Thus it is one of a very long list of diseases that may be said to be caused by humans, by sins of omission rather than commission. We know how to prevent outbreaks, but in these cases we failed to do so.

Possibly the most extreme examples of such sins occurred in the 19th and 20th centuries, in the form of concentration camps and the Irish potato famine. The concentration camps might have been specifically dreamt up by warped scientists as a means of establishing the optimum conditions for establishing epidemics. Indeed, Nazi 'doctors' actually carried out some research, including deliberate inoculation of diseases like malaria into human subjects, in the hope of discovering a vaccine. For the most part, though, the Nazis' 'Final Solution' of eradicating the races they considered inferior, so reminiscent of a strain of bacteria attempting to control an ecological niche, included infectious diseases almost by accident.

We need to beware of holocaust-denying revisionism in examining the statistics about the deaths of concentration camp inmates. There are those who would have us believe the deaths were almost an accident, but there is no doubt that epidemic infectious disease, in the form of typhus, relapsing fever, diarrhoeal illness and tuberculosis, was responsible for a high proportion of them. Here is the evidence as presented by Jan Sehn, the judge who presided over the Auschwitz trials in Poland, in his report *Concentration Camp Oswiecim-Brzezinka* (Auschwitz-Birkenau).

None of the camp huts had ventilation. The floor was of clay, which during droughts, clouds of dust would rise, while during wet weather a large puddle would form where the roof leaked. In these conditions, the huts were a breeding place for fleas, lice and rats, which plagued the inmates and carried infectious diseases ... Lice infection, scabies and mange, as well as violent epidemics of typhus which decimated the prisoners especially in winter, were the inevitable consequences of the anti-humanitarian hygienic and sanitary conditions in the camp. They inexorably followed the lack of water, the impossibility of washing and changing underclothes, and the incredible overcrowding in huts ... the prisoners were also decimated by typhoid fever in all its varieties, and by malaria ... The starved and undermined constitutions of the inmates were incapable of resistance to disease, and the death rate among the sick was very high.

You would struggle to invent a better breeding ground for human disease than malnourished, stressed and overworked men and women in overcrowded, unhygienic conditions, whose numbers were replenished frequently by trainloads of fresh victims carrying new diseases.

Similar charges may be laid at the feet of the responsible authorities following the Irish potato famine. While it may not be true that this was the consequence of an act of deliberate genocide, there is no doubt that many in authority considered the Irish an inferior race. Relief for famine victims (although not completely absent) was dilatory and inadequate. As a result it could be argued that it is as inaccurate to include this among the 'natural disasters' as it is concentration camps. Subsequent epidemics of louse-borne typhus and relapsing fever caused further misery to the displaced masses, who were often evicted from their homes. Nor was there much relief for those who emigrated; travelling on starvation rations many died of typhus in ships across the Atlantic, or in quarantine once they arrived. Mortality in the so-called 'coffin ships' arriving in Canada was in the order of 20 per cent. Like bacterial spores they carried the diseases with them, and epidemics of typhus in British North America (Canada) and the United States followed. Thus we are an epidemic in this sense, through our inhumanity.

The Four Horsemen of the Apocalypse in the title of this chapter are, of course, pestilence, war, famine and death. They ride together. As the great bacteriologist Zinsser wrote in 1937 in *Rats, Lice and History*, 'soldiers have rarely won wars. They more often mop up after the barrage of epidemics.' Up to the end of the 19th century typhus, cholera and dysentery conventionally killed more soldiers than enemy action. Such conflicts sometimes send out ripples and whirlpools far away from their centres; as was the case with Maria.

Maria's story

Maria arrived at our hospital through an unusual route. She had been involved in a fight outside a department store and had been injured. In fact, she had been struck over the side of her head so violently that her eardrum was perforated. She was arrested. After a little while it became clear that she was confused. It took some time to discover this because her English was poor. She had recently arrived in England and her native language was Spanish; she had escaped from a war zone as a refugee. The police doctor was called to assess her injuries and found that she had a high fever. As a consequence, she was sent to our hospital and this is where we encountered her.

There was very little of real significance to find when she was examined; she had some blood on her head and face at the site of her injury. Her temperature was recorded at an elevated 39 degrees. A clue to the diagnosis was that her pulse rate was barely elevated at 90 beats per minute. Conventionally fever means a rapid pulse as the body seeks to cool itself by increasing flow through the smaller blood vessels which act like radiators. There are, though, a few illnesses where this normal response does not occur. We put her on antibiotics with a view to treating the illness we suspected, while we waited for laboratory confirmation the next day.

Modern culture of human blood for bacteria takes place in sophisticated machines. These are both incubators and detectors. When there is active living material in the blood it consumes oxygen and releases carbon dioxide as a by-product. When this happens the acidity in the blood suspension changes, and this causes a shift in the colour of an indicator in the bottle. Electronic sensors constantly monitor the colour of the indicator. When it changes, an alarm is sounded and the bottle is removed for examination. At this point much older technology is resorted to. The blood is smeared on a slide and stained with artificial dyes. This is known as the Gram stain, and is one of the oldest methods available in microbiology. It remains as useful today as it was when invented by Hans Christian Gram in 1882.

The test of Maria's blood showed that it was teeming with bacilli. They absorbed the stain in a manner typical of the organisms known as Gram-negative. This gave us a broad early clue about the nature of the bacterium that was poisoning her. Our early suspicions were confirmed. Maria had typhoid.

The hateful vaccine

We see typhoid rarely in the West nowadays. Such cases as there are tend to be imported from countries where sewage arrangements are rudimentary, or disrupted by natural disaster or conflict. The bacterium is transmitted primarily in faeces, and thus in contaminated water. Once it was among the foremost among our killers, and it is said to have carried off Schubert, William the Conqueror and both of Pasteur's daughters. Typhoid and cholera are the diseases that were vanquished in Britain by Sir Joseph Bazalgette and his sewerage system, as well as by the brilliant but dogmatic Almwroth Wright, who developed the first vaccine. He offered it to soldiers serving in the Boer War, who promptly threw the cases of vaccine overboard as the ships sailed from their British harbours. It made them feel ill, they said.

Of the British Force of 556,653 men who served in the Anglo-Boer War, 57,684 contracted typhoid, 8,225 of whom died, while 7,582 were killed in action. The vaccine was taken up by the War Office for the First World War. The mortality from typhoid fell so abruptly that only about 2,000 British troops died from the disease in the entire conflict.

The image of soldiers throwing an unpopular vaccine overboard in 1899 to their own detriment is a potent one for our times. It is an early, prophetic echo of the superstitious and misguided suspicions about modern vaccines. This is the earliest example of a phenomenon that has become widespread. As has been stated, the polio vaccine is being rejected in some countries. In some parts of Britain, as a result of inaccurate scare stories about its possible dangers, the uptake of MMR fell to below 75 per cent, while in order to ensure that the disease cannot spread, an uptake of greater than 95 per cent is required. The United Kingdom reported its first death for years from measles in 2006.

In the Republic of Ireland in 2000, the low uptake of the combined vaccine resulted in an outbreak of 1,220 cases of measles and the deaths of three children. In the Netherlands in 1999–2000, a religious community that refuses vaccination had a measles epidemic of over 2,300 cases. Almost 20 per cent had serious complications, and three children died. This is the other kind of epidemic that troubles humans: one of superstition and disregard for the informed opinion of qualified experts. This is the sense in which we are epidemics in the same way that the soldiers of the Boer War were. They were carried off by the fifth and sixth horsemen, arrogance and ignorance.

We shall now move on to consider an epidemic which is, at first sight, unrelated to infectious disease. That is the dramatic increase in diseases of allergy in the western world. As we shall see, there is more than a tangential connection between infection and allergy. This may also apply to more sinister diseases, and even to cancers.

CHAPTER 7

THE AUTO-IMMUNITY
AND CANCER EPIDEMIC

The western world faces an entirely new and terrifying variety
of epidemic, and one that is not apparently infectious. While
the developing world still suffers all the traditional epidemics of
tuberculosis, malaria and cholera, we are struggling with at least
one that may be caused by affluence. The number of people
living with asthma, allergies and hayfever has reached almost
pandemic proportions.

For example, the number of admissions to hospitals in
England and Wales for anaphylaxis (the most severe, life-threatening form of allergy) has increased by 600 per cent since 1990,
and admissions for food allergy are up by 400 per cent. Consul-
tations with family doctors for hayfever increased by 260 per
cent between 1971 and 1991. Although the trend for asthma may
have stabilised in recent years, there is no doubt that all western
nations have seen a huge increase in the number of new sufferers, and from a disease that can kill.

Food that can kill

A colleague of mine has a daughter who has a severe food allergy; in her case it is to nuts. This is an increasingly common condition, and kills several children a year, almost exclusively in the West. The really horrible feature of this incurable condition is that as time goes by each allergic reaction to nuts is worse than the last. Many allergies can be cured by gradual 'desensitisation' with initially tiny but gradually increasing doses of the trigger cause. This has been tried in nut allergy, but tragically with fatal results.

I remember having Mike and his family for lunch one Sunday. We knew about the problem; we were certain not to include any nuts in the food we planned to offer his daughter. We provided the child with some ice cream instead of the apple crumble we were all eating. She borrowed her sister's spoon to eat it. Just in time her mother knocked the spoon from her fingers. She had noticed that we had used almonds in the crumble mix, and even the amount present on a used spoon might have been enough to trigger a fatal reaction.

A peculiarity of this epidemic of allergies is that it seems to be taking place principally in the parts of the world where we had infectious diseases on the back foot. In countries still ravaged by the old infectious enemies, asthma, hayfever and similar diseases are far more rare. There could be many explanations for this; perhaps it could be a genetic, racial predisposition. Air pollution has been mooted as a possible cause, as have central heating and carpets. But there are other explanations that fit the facts more closely, and these explanations bring us once again to my central premise, that we are epidemics.

A disease of the rich

An intriguing observation has been that genetically similar peoples around the Baltic Sea – Scandinavians on the one side, Latvians, Estonians and Lithuanians on the other – traditionally had differing rates of asthma. Such diseases were far more common in the more westernised nations of Sweden, Denmark and Norway. Then, relatively abruptly, the situation began to change. Following the fall of communist domination in the nations of the Baltic, rates of allergic disease began to rise.

This is the sort of epidemic that seems to fit with an infectious cause. However, although it was widely believed up to this point that an individual asthma episode might be triggered by infection, the notion that infectious disease might underlie the entire condition had not even been considered. Explanations of the kind mentioned above – central heating, pollution and so forth – simply did not seem to fit the facts in this case, though. Some scientists began to explore another hypothesis, and to challenge some assumptions about the origins of allergy.

Let us consider asthma first. The conventional hypothesis works something like this. The passages and airways that allow air to flow through our lungs are variable in diameter. This makes physiological sense; it may be necessary to increase the airflow when we exercise and reduce it when we are at rest. The calibre of these tubes is altered by circular muscles which surround them. These muscles are, like all muscles, under the control of nerves. Such nerves are not like those that tell our arms and legs to move, they are more like the nerves of our intestines, and they operate without our conscious control.

All of these nerves of the so-called autonomic nervous system are under the influence of chemicals like adrenaline. They are also influenced by other chemicals called cytokines, which are produced by white blood cells. In asthma, in response to an inhaled trigger, the white blood cells produce too much of the cytokine and the muscles go into spasm. The allergen that acts as the trigger might be inhaled pollen, or fungal spores, or house dust mites, or one of a number of substances capable of exciting the same response including foods. Other allergies basically obey the same mechanism; an overproduction of cytokines by white blood cells causes a local reaction in the skin, or the intestine, or the nose.

The particular white blood cells responsible for producing these cytokines are known as eosinophils, on the basis that they are identified by their absorption of a synthetic stain called eosin. The major cytokine they produce is histamine; anti-histamines are of course a standard treatment for allergies. They do so in conjunction with another product of white blood cells, which is an immunoglobulin. These are proteins which regulate the immune response, and the particular variety we are interested in here is called Immunoglobulin E, or IgE for short. In broad terms immunoglobulins serve the function of 'flagging up' foreign material for attack.

Very little happens in nature without an evolutionary reason behind it. At first glance it may seem nonsensical to have a branch of immunity which only seems to cause misery in the form of breathlessness, wheeze, itchy skin rash and runny noses. However, when the principal function of the IgE/eosinophil/histamine response is revealed then a possible clue to the dramatic emergence of the asthma/hayfever epidemic emerges. Eosinophils are responsible for combating one of the great historical burdens of humankind, the parasites. In particular they mobilise immune responses to tapeworms and illnesses caused by larvae. These are conditions rarely encountered in the West; although children still sometimes contract roundworms (the principal symptom of which is, interestingly given the symptoms of allergy, itch), we are largely free nowadays of the massive burden of worms which still trouble the developing world, as discussed in Chapter 4.

This, then, is the hypothesis, and it is known as the hygiene hypothesis for reasons that will become obvious. Human social evolution has overtaken biological evolution. We are able to control our environment to such a degree that we are no longer exposed to the same infectious challenges. Clean drinking water and regulation of food handling have eradicated many of the scourges of the past, such as typhoid, cholera and tapeworms. We are paying a price, though. We have a branch of our immunity that is at a 'loose end'. When it encounters something even vaguely resembling its natural target, it goes into overdrive and produces cytokines and IgE in quantities that cause the familiar symptoms of asthma and allergy.

What is worse, the usual trigger for shutdown of the armed response has been lost. Normally, when an infection is controlled, the signal to terminate the immune response is the eradication of the infection itself. This is important, because in many infections – tuberculosis for example, and hepatitis B – it is the immune reaction that causes damage rather than toxic products of the infection itself. Thus the immune response needs to be told when to switch off, otherwise uncontrolled damage could result.

Why, then, did the fall of the Iron Curtain contribute to the rising incidence of asthma and allergy in the old soviet Baltic states? One theory is that economic realities simply changed at that moment, and with them human behaviour. Previously the model for agriculture was the collective farm. State control of the means of production meant that many people supplemented their food supplies with small-scale cultivation in their own gardens. A substantial proportion of the population had some regular contact with soil and the land, often from an early age. With economic liberalisation and the advent of a more capitalist market model, many simply ceased this habit and bought their vegetables from supermarkets, packaged, cleaned and shrink-wrapped, just like in the West.

The tapeworm, our friend

It is not only asthma and allergies that may be related to the hygiene hypothesis, and we have discussed elsewhere (in Chapter 4) how insects may cure patients. There are those who now believe that tapeworms may have therapeutic value in other diseases. Dr Joel Weinstock and his colleagues from the University of Iowa has claimed (in the *New Scientist*) that regular doses of certain worms (*Trichuris trichuria*) might cure people with inflammatory bowel diseases such as ulcerative colitis and Crohn's disease. Such diseases are increasingly common in the developed world; Weinstock believes it is because we are no longer exposed to parasites. Dr Weinstock has treated six patients by introducing into their bowels eggs which hatched, developing into parasitic worms. Five of the six patients – who had failed conventional treatment – went into complete remission.

In an even more exciting piece of research, a team from Britain, led by Dr Anne Cooke of the Pathology Department of Cambridge University, has made the amazing discovery that diabetes may be prevented in mice if they are infected with the parasite *Schistosoma*, the agent of bilharzia. This was an entirely serendipitous discovery. When she moved her laboratory, mice bred to develop Type 1 diabetes for research purposes accidentally became exposed to the parasite. The expectation was that 80 per cent of the mice would develop diabetes; the reality was 50 per cent.

The team repeated the experiment with younger mice exposed to the schistosome eggs; this time none developed diabetes. The finding correlates with the observation that populations with a high incidence of schistosomiasis have a low incidence of diabetes. It seemed to be the egg itself that had the effect, rather than the later, older stages of the parasite. The team is now hot on the trail of the precise substance present in the egg that causes the effect. It would then be possible to administer that harmless substance without causing bilharzia, and prevent diabetes. If the hygiene hypothesis is ultimately proven, then there is no reason that the same principle should not apply to illnesses like asthma, rheumatoid arthritis and inflammatory bowel disease, which share some causes with diabetes in being auto-immune.

Sean's story ...

The concept of damage to our bodies from the body's own misdirected response to infection is well established in medical science. I well remember a child called Sean, whom we were asked to see by our colleagues in the department of paediatrics at our hospital. Sean was an identical age and of very similar appearance to my own son; every time I visited him I found my silent will for him to recover was almost palpable. Objectivity in medicine is not always easy.

Sean had become acutely unwell with a very high fever, severe headache and a widespread rash all over his body. The rash was unusual in that it spared the area around his mouth, which remained pale. Not so the folds of his skin at his wrists, elbows and knees, which were a deep, livid red. His tongue had an evil-looking yellowish coating, with bright red spots of normal tongue poking through. The skin was slightly roughened to the touch, almost like very fine sandpaper. The poor lad was extremely ill at first. His blood pressure had dropped sufficiently to require replacement of intravenous fluid. His mother was terrified.

Sean's description would be almost instantly recognisable to most older physicians. The diagnosis was once far commoner than it is now. In the severe toxic form in which Sean had the illness, it has become very rare. The disease is scarlet fever, and it is caused by an organism called *Streptococcus pyogenes*, also known as Group A Streptococcus. The particular strain of the organism that Sean had caught was able to produce a poison, the so-called erythrogenic toxin. With skilled treatment he recovered fully, and I was delighted when he left the hospital fit and well, in time for Christmas. However, not everyone who encounters the Group A streptococcus is quite so lucky.

... and Norman's

In another ward of the same hospital was an affable, charming white-haired elderly gentleman called Norman. Had I encountered him 68 years ago his appearance would have been almost identical to Sean's. He too had had scarlet fever. Now, though, he was suffering the consequences of that brush with this very dangerous bug. Unlike Sean he had not been treated with antibiotics for the disease, and had progressed to a very serious complication, acute rheumatic fever. This is one of a number of complications that can be caused by infection with the Group A Streptococcus. Put simply, to the immune system, substances on the surface of some strains of the bacterium closely resemble human tissue. There then follows a case of mistaken identity. The body's immune response ceases to identify its own tissue as 'self' and begins to attack it. This is known as molecular mimicry. Some tissues are more susceptible than others, presumably because they carry markers on them which are particularly akin to *Streptococcus pyogenes*. These are the tissues of the heart, brain and kidney.

Norman's heart had suffered in this particular bout. He had been left with damaged valves, and this had led to our encounter with him. He had developed fatigue, breathlessness and anaemia, with a slight fever and sweating at night. A simple ultrasound test showed large suspicious clots on his heart valves. We obtained specimens of his blood, which confirmed that a different species of streptococcus was the cause. The bacteria had begun to adhere to the damaged tissue of his heart. Norman had the same disease that had killed Gustav Mahler, endocarditis.

Norman was not to be as lucky as Sean. Proper cure of endocarditis requires prolonged treatment in hospital with intravenous antibiotics and sometimes even heart surgery. The poor old gentleman was condemned to spend one his few remaining Christmases in the lugubrious and functional surroundings of a British National Health Service medical ward.

This syndrome of late damage to tissues following an acute infection with streptococci is a classical variant, familiar to every medical student. Although it has been well described, the syndromes like Norman and Sean's are rare. In fact *Streptococcus pyogenes* is no longer as dangerous as it once was, for reasons that are not fully understood by the scientific community. However, as scientific knowledge advances it has become clear that many conditions arise from the same cause, and that some of these diseases are very common indeed, to the point of being epidemic in proportions.

Failure of the pancreas

Diabetes mellitus is extremely common in affluent, well-nourished nations; it occurs in about one in 200 people, and the incidence is increasing. It is an incurable condition where the cells of the pancreas responsible for producing insulin simply die, attacked by the body's own immune cells. For simplicity's sake I am concentrating here on the Type 1 sort of diabetes; there is another, Type 2, sort, which generally appears later in life and is associated with obesity. The consequence of both is that sugar is not properly metabolised and toxic products accumulate in body tissues. These can cause kidney failure, heart disease, blindness and greater susceptibility to infection. It is not at all a pleasant condition. Replacement of the natural insulin by artificial insulin controls the disease and saves lives, but is unfortunately not curative.

The concept that an infection may trigger diabetes is not a new one. Any condition that damages the pancreas may lead to diabetes; this includes trauma, alcohol abuse, scorpion bites and the viral infection mumps. Clues that another, less obvious infection may be partly responsible began to appear in the 1990s, when viral particles were isolated in the pancreas of a child dying from diabetes. The particular virus was identified as belonging to the enteroviruses, and is known as Coxsackie B4. The Coxsackie family are named after a town in the state of New York; the virus was first discovered in 1948 in that town by researchers investigating the polio virus, to which it is related.

This family of viruses is responsible for a long list of conditions, including some that can cause epidemics in their own right. The island of Bornholm in Denmark was once wracked by an epidemic of lower chest pain resembling heart attacks. Coxsackie B4 was found to be the cause of that condition, which is also known as the Devil's Grip. The same virus is now well established as a key cause of diabetes.

Almost certainly you will have encountered Coxsackie viruses; you may well have been infected with Coxsackie B4. They are extremely common and widespread, and most adults have evidence of infection at some time in their lives in the form of antibodies. Yet not every person who is infected with B4 ends up with diabetes. Why is this so?

The answer is that a further factor is required. To contract *diabetes mellitus* following a viral infection, you have to be the right kind of individual by virtue of your inheritance. You need to have exactly the right constellation of genes. This is a common feature in auto-immune conditions, and there are others.

Nick's story

Nick was 23 years old. The nurse who brought his case notes in commented how strikingly good-looking and charming he was; she suggested that his mere attendance in the out-patients department had 'made her day'. He was a university student, and by his own admission was 'popular with the ladies'. When I encountered him, though, he was feeling a little sorry for himself. He had developed very sore eyes, a sore back, feet and ankles, and an agonising burning pain in the tip of his penis on passing urine.

We had no difficulty at all in establishing a diagnosis; in fact my colleague who had referred him to us even included the possible diagnosis in the accompanying letter. Nick had Reiter's syndrome. Given his lifestyle it was reasonable to suppose that his was a complication of infection with the bacterium *Chlamydia trachomatis*. Nick confessed that he had had this common sexually acquired infection a few weeks previously. I would have bet a fair sum of money that I could have predicted his genetic make-up. Nick had an 80 per cent chance of carrying a gene called HLA B27.

Nick's arthritis, conjunctivitis and urethritis responded to anti-inflammatory drugs. Reiter's is not a common illness, and certainly does not fit any useful definition of an epidemic. Auto-immune diseases as a general category are increasingly common, however, with up to 8 per cent of the population suffering from one, 78 per cent of these being women. They are the third most common group of diseases in the United States after heart disease and cancer; between 14 and 22 million people are said to be affected. Some are very common indeed. The list of auto-immune conditions believed to be associated with a triggering infection is quite a long one, and includes one of the world's most common disabling diseases, rheumatoid arthritis.

The mimics

However, I have introduced the concept of genetic susceptibility to long-term consequences of an infection for other reasons, which are crucial to epidemics. The first is that auto-immunity is not wholly a negative phenomenon. I referred above to the concept of molecular mimicry, whereby the body is 'tricked' into attacking itself by a microbe which has constituents apparently identical to that of its victim. There is another mechanism whereby auto-immunity may arise. Viruses attack the body in quite a different way from bacteria, parasites or other agents of epidemics. They do so by hijacking the machinery of the victim's cell and using it to reproduce. In doing so they must, by necessity, enter the cell itself. Viruses then take the process a stage further, incorporating their genes into the chromosomes of the host. The body is then presented with a real challenge – to destroy the invader while not destroying itself. In contrast bacteria can and do invade human and animal cells in order to cause disease, but they do not incorporate their genetic material into the host's, which makes them easier to attack.

A cell that has been invaded by a virus will change. Because the virus' genes are translated into proteins, some of which will be used to make new copies of the virus, some will form envelopes for the virus to be a complete product, but some will appear on the surface of the cell itself. This forms the basis of the body's response to infected cells. The alien proteins on their surface will serve as triggers for destruction by the body's own defences. Thus, some viral infections can cause an auto-immune response. The actual damage to the tissues is not caused by the virus, but by the toxic response to it.

Harry's story

One patient sticks very clearly in my mind as a victim of this phenomenon. Harry noticed one day while he was shaving that his eyes had changed colour – the usual clear whites had changed to a sickly yellow. He had been unwell for a few days, with pains in his joints and a general feeling of just not being right. He was a pharmacist, and had no difficulty in recognising that he was jaundiced. He had also noticed that his urine had become dark, almost the colour of black coffee. He made an emergency appointment to see his family doctor, and within a few hours was admitted to our hospital.

Diagnosis of the common causes of jaundice relies on a few straightforward tests. Characteristic enzyme patterns in the blood will reveal whether the problem is an obstruction to the flow of bile, and simple radiography will confirm or refute this. Harry's blood tests showed that he had hepatitis, and there was no suggestion that his bile duct was blocked. Most causes of hepatitis require no treatment, so at first we simply observed him while we awaited the results of the tests that would tell us which of the alphabetical list of viruses it was likely to be; hepatitis A, B, C, D or E.

Had I been a betting man, at this point I would have put my money on A. My reasoning was that the way Harry lived his life – we had asked about this in detail – made B, C and D unlikely. These viruses are transmitted by blood-to-blood contact, which generally happens through needle sharing, transfusion of blood, sex or some kind of accident. Harry's life appeared risk-free in this respect. A and E are ingested with contaminated food or water, but E does not often occur in Britain, and Harry had not travelled within the incubation period. Hepatitis A, although uncommon in western countries, does occur. At this stage we were quite relaxed about the outcome – A rarely kills.

I can recall the exact moment when the laboratory rang me with the result. One of my colleagues was teaching medical students, using Harry as a living teaching aid. I knew instantly that I would have to subtly, discreetly inform my doctor friend about Harry's diagnosis and interrupt the flow of education. Clinicians need to be aware that the patient they are instructing students on carries a blood-borne, infectious virus. Even though the students should have been vaccinated, risk management dictates that precautions must be taken. Harry had hepatitis B. I passed a hurriedly scribbled note to my colleague via a nurse who pretended to be checking his medications chart.

I returned later in the day to ask Harry some more questions. Patients are sometimes embarrassed to confess to sexual encounters or other perceived misdemeanours; gentle persistence can often pay off. This is not just prurience, since uncovering risky behaviour can help prevent future infections. On one occasion we were able to identify a tattoo parlour where the needles were not being properly sterilised.

The incubation period for hepatitis B is 30–120 days, so we talked carefully through Harry's life over that period. He was a sexually abstinent bachelor. His claim that he had never experimented with any drug stronger than dry sherry was readily credible. The only possible hint of a risk was an apparently trivial incident that he had almost forgotten. A couple of months earlier a young man with a bleeding hand had come into his pharmacy to buy sticking plasters. Harry, a naturally kind and helpful soul, had cleaned the wound and applied the plaster for him.

This gentle act might have been his undoing. Hepatitis B is transmissible in microscopic, invisible quantities of blood. Some tiny break in Harry's own skin – and he was a keen gardener – could readily have let the deadly virus in.

Over the following days we watched in alarm as his liver deteriorated. It became apparent that he was developing fulminant hepatic failure, a complication of hepatitis B. We enlisted the assistance of our colleagues the hepatologists. Harry required the very best treatment then available, including a spell in the intensive care department. He very nearly died. This episode occurred some years ago; it is possible that nowadays he might even have been considered for a liver transplant. Although Harry had had some terrible bad luck, he had the good fortune to survive.

Hepatitis B may be considered an epidemic disease. In the United States alone there are 300,000 new infections per year, with 300 deaths from acute liver failure. A further 4,000–5,000 die from cirrhosis or liver cancer as a consequence of chronic infection. In some countries such as New Guinea and the Solomon Islands, where transmission occurs from infected mother to baby or in early childhood, up to 50 per cent of 10 to 20-year-olds can be shown by blood testing to have been exposed to the virus. However, I am exploring hepatitis B here for a different reason.

The damage that occurred to Harry's liver arose not entirely as a result of toxins produced by the virus itself, but because his own immune response vigorously annihilated the cells that carried the markers of infection. This is not an uncommon feature of epidemic diseases. The great influenza pandemic of 1918–20 killed so many for much the same reason. Indeed, the fact that so many younger people died reflected the vigour of their immune systems. Auto-immunity as a cause of tissue damage occurs in many other viral infections, including HIV/AIDS and hepatitis C, as well as bacterial diseases such as tuberculosis, leprosy and Lyme disease.

Our variant genes

The same cells of the immune response are responsible for auto-immune diseases as are responsible for tissue damage in tuberculosis. There has been a slightly less scientific observation that people with auto-immune disease rarely contract tuberculosis. These two pieces of information have led scientists to look at the genes that confer resistance to tuberculosis, and susceptibility to auto-immune disease.

The results of these investigations have been startling. Susceptibility to tuberculosis may be conferred by rogue genes encoding a cytokine called TNF-alpha, which is a vital chemical in combating the infection. There are a number of different variants of the gene. People who have variant 308A are more susceptible than average to the auto-immune diseases lupus, rheumatoid arthritis, and another auto-immune disease principally affecting the eye called Sjogren's syndrome. Those who have the 308GG variant (people cannot have both this and 308A) are more susceptible to tuberculosis. It is now strongly suspected that these genes represent two sides of the same coin. Genes that confer resistance to tuberculosis also make people susceptible to auto-immunity, and vice versa. In other words an epidemic of auto-immunity is the price we have paid as a species for resistance to infectious epidemics.

The actual mechanics of how we begin to attack ourselves and cause these peculiar illnesses may be even more bizarre and unexpected. Elsewhere in this book we encountered human endogenous retroviruses (HERVs). They are discussed more fully in the chapter concerning viruses, but I shall recap briefly here. Some of what follows is necessarily somewhat dense and scientific. I have tried to express it clearly and to use analogies, but to fully understand how much human existence is defined by infectious disease we must follow it through. I should emphasise that the science of the study of HERVs is in its relative infancy. Much of what follows is speculative but based on compelling evidence.

HERVs are genetic sequences found in our chromosomes that are unquestionably viral remnants, suggesting that these viruses infected us long ago in our evolutionary history. They are almost identical in structure and nature to the agent of AIDS, HIV. They differ in that they are immortalised in our genes, and are passed on from parent to offspring. They comprise a startling 8 per cent of our genes. You do not have to catch a HERV, you are born with them. Retroviruses that are acquired in life are known as exogenous retroviruses (XRVs). Our evolutionary ancestors acquired XRVs, and either because they were useful, or because it was too costly in energy to expel them, they stuck and became HERVs. Most are believed to be about 20–40 million years old, although some are older, and some younger. They are rather like the ancient foundations of a modern city which has been rebuilt many times over; long since forgotten, they have nevertheless served, and continue to serve, a vital function.

Most HERVs are inactive, most of the time. They are simply not translated into proteins. Some products of HERVs are translated into useful proteins, though – syncitin, for instance, which helps our cells to stick to one another. The best example of a HERV with a known function is HERV-W. The proteins of this HERV are vital for an essential step during formation of the placenta and are thus vital for our survival as a species. There are even those who believe that the development of human consciousness relied upon the properties of HERVs. The evidence for this comes from fruit flies, where some endogenous retroviruses (ERVs) produce a sudden increase in the complexity and quantity of nerve material.

Proteins are sequences of amino acids. If you know the sequence, it is relatively easy to deduce the gene sequence that encoded it. Once you have unravelled the protein, predicting the genetic sequence is really no harder than deriving a house address by using the post or zip code, although repeated many times over. From such patterns it is possible to deduce which proteins we are dealing with that are encoded by HERVs.

It is then possible to look at HERV-encoded proteins that appear in disease but not in health. There are further layers of sophistication. To encode a protein, DNA must first be transcribed into RNA; it is possible to examine the RNA sequences for HERV products. It is also possible to look for evidence of HERVs in the form of antibodies. There is, though, a serious limitation to the science. This is really 'guilt by association'. The usual rules for proving that any agent causes an infectious disease are the Koch postulates (see page 148), where the agent must be introduced into a species and then cause disease. Clearly this is not possible where the virus is already permanently present in the chromosomes.

In animals it is possible to breed strains that have ERVs deleted, and to look at the impact on diseases, but this is not feasible or desirable in humans. There are variations in human inheritance of HERVs which can be examined, but beyond that there is little more than a statistical association of HERVs and disease, and a plausible scientific explanation.

How ERVs might cause disease

That explanation is really two-fold. ERVs may cause disease by suddenly becoming active and producing toxic products, or by shifting genes around in the chromosomes, or both. Retroviruses rely on moving DNA about to survive – they have to do so in order to incorporate themselves into the host and ultimately escape. This is essential to their nature, and is a property which has been 'tamed' in inactive HERVs. However, they can suddenly become 'un-tame', through mutation or some other trigger. If they do so, they may move to a different part of the chromosome, where they become active.

To pursue our 'ancient city foundations' analogy, it is as though a bit of Roman wall under the City of London suddenly gives way and causes a modern building to collapse. The analogy would be even more exact if those Roman foundations were moved by an incompetent builder or blown up by a terrorist's bomb. When the HERV genes activate, they will by necessity nearly but not precisely resemble human proteins. They will also have escaped the process that all of us undergo early in life, where our cells are 'checked' by immunity to ensure that what is us and what is not us is clearly demarcated. Thus they are excellent candidates for 'molecular mimicry', where the body attacks itself because it confuses its own proteins with those of an invader.

Schizophrenia, multiple sclerosis, gomerulonephritis, systemic lupus erythematosus, diabetes and rheumatoid arthritis are all diseases that have, or are believed to have, an auto-immune component. In each there has been evidence of altered expression of HERV proteins or RNA. That is not the same as saying these components cause the disease, as is explained above, but they are consistently present at the scene of the crime. It is also not a complete explanation. Why do some people develop these diseases when all of us have HERVs, and basically the same ones? What makes them 'un-tame'? Mutation is one possibility, as has been said. Another is genetic variability in other parts of our chromosomes. A further viral infection is another, as with our Coxsackie example in diabetes. This certainly seems plausible in the case of HERVs and cancers, discussed below.

It would be a logical extension of this argument that 'un-tamed' XRVs like HIV (those acquired during our own lifetimes) should also cause auto-immune disease. This is unquestionably the case. The list of reported auto-immune diseases in HIV/AIDS includes systemic lupus erythematosus, anti-phospholipid syndrome, vasculitis, primary biliary cirrhosis, polymyositis, Graves' disease and idiopathic thrombocytopenic purpura.

Another retrovirus that infects humans – HTLV-1, a cause of leukaemia in some parts of the world – is associated with an auto-immune disease of the thyroid gland, and probably others. I do not propose to detail the precise clinical manifestations of this long list of diseases, but I hope I have made the point. Retroviruses, whether they are encoded in our chromosomes or acquired in life, are powerfully associated with auto-immune diseases. Their association is supported by a convincing scientific rationale. We suffer these diseases because we are composed of epidemic material. Once again, we are epidemics.

The western world is also in the grip of two further epidemics: heart disease and cancer. We shall come back to heart disease, but first we shall look at cancer and infection.

What causes cancer

The association between cancer and infection has long been known. There is a list of viruses that are known to cause cancer. They include Epstein Barr virus (the cause of glandular fever, which can lead to a variety of cancers including lymphoma), human papilloma virus (cervical cancer), human herpes virus type 8 (Kaposi's sarcoma), and hepatitis B and C (hepatocellular carcinoma). Nor are viruses exclusively the cause. Chronic infection with the parasite *Schistosoma* is causative in bladder cancer, and the fluke *Chlonorchis sinensis* is strongly associated with some kinds of liver cancer. There is some evidence that lung cancer may be more common in people who have had pulmonary tuberculosis, even if it has been cured. However, these links, although fascinating in their own right, do not make up the main thrust of my argument.

Although 'cancer' is one of the world's major killers, especially in the West, it is an umbrella term and includes many, many different diagnoses. One interpretation of the epidemic of cancer in developed nations is that freedom from infectious diseases permits us to live long enough to have the 'luxury' of dying from it in later life. After all, we all have to die of something.

At the heart of the definition of 'cancer', though, are two basic principles, one a sort of accelerator, the other a failure of the brakes. The 'accelerator' is the loss of the regulation of the growth process of cells. This means that a single variety, or clone, of cells proliferates without restraint. The 'brake failure' is a flaw in surveillance of these abnormally reproducing cells. Essentially this means that our immunity normally recognises aberrant and defective cells and eradicates them. In the cancerous state, somehow the abnormal cells evade the detection and destruction of immunity. An excellent example of this is in HIV/AIDS. The cells that are principally destroyed by HIV are T-lymphocytes, whose principal task is to recognise abnormal tissue and flag it up for destruction. In advanced AIDS, when there are very few of these lymphocytes remaining, the risk of developing some kinds of cancer increases massively.

At a superficial level this disturbance of proliferation and regulation has much in common with an infection. Bacteria reproduce and proliferate as clones, like cancer cells, restricted only by their access to nutrients and their own toxic waste products. In a successful infection, like cancer cells they are capable of evading the immune response and preventing their own identification and destruction. Indeed, some infections are believed to cause cancer by persistent and long-term thwarting of an effective immune response, as the confused and chronically inflamed immune cells lose their own regulation and themselves become cancerous. This is believed to be the mechanism of gall bladder cancer in liver fluke (Clonorchis) infection.

Viral infection is even more closely related to cancers, in that both depend on alterations to the genes of the victim. Viral genes become incorporated into the DNA of the host in order to reproduce; that is an essential part of their life cycle. In order for cells to become cancerous, their genes must encode the capacity for unrestricted proliferation, as was mentioned above. The gene that encodes for this may be introduced by a viral infection.

This explains both why some viruses cause cancer, and why environmental factors like ionising radiation that stimulate gene mutation have the same effect. The presence of the viral abnormal cancer-causing gene may not rely wholly on infection during the life of the victim. ERVs are implicated here. Their capacity to cause cancer in animals is incontrovertible. One of the first ERVs ever described is also known as mouse mammary tumour virus (MMTV), which as its name suggests causes cancer in mice. This virus can exist in two forms. One is the infectious variant identical to other viruses, and the other is permanently encoded into species of mouse and present in all offspring.

There is mounting evidence that the same may be true in humans. There are certainly infectious retroviruses that can cause cancer (HTLV-1 causes adult T-cell leukaemia), and there are certainly ERVs that appear to be implicated in the development of cancer. The most convincing to date is the cancer called the seminoma, which is a variety of testicular cancer. Other candidates are malignant melanoma and breast cancer. Although it is by no means 100 per cent proven that ERVs 'cause' cancer at present, it seems increasingly clear that they are involved at some level. A likely theory is that some ERVs provide a mechanism for causing cancer, and that a further trigger – probably another viral infection – is required to activate it. I shall stick my neck out a little and say that it is likely that other cancers will turn out to have an ERV association.

Here, then, is another sense in which humans 'are' epidemics, and that is through our susceptibility to cancer. There is no question that a significant proportion of our genes arose from infection with these ERVs. Harbouring them can have a range of effects, from beneficial to neutral to dangerous. Nevertheless within the very essence of our being we *are* ERVs, and a possible consequence of that is the risk of developing cancer.

Evolution is, almost by definition, a trade-off between benefit and risk in acquiring genes. Some ERVs have been shown to encode useful products vital to our survival. The majority of cancers arise later in life; at least, the risk of developing cancer increases with age. Thus cancer does not necessarily reduce the reproductive capacity of our species. From the perspective of the selfish gene, then, it is a sort of irrelevance, and it is 'worth' acquiring the risk along with the benefits of ERVs.

Struggle and adaptation

At a further, more philosophical level, the tendency of our cells to become deregulated and cancerous is also a product of our struggle with epidemics. If we faced no infectious challenge, we would require far less adaptability within our cells. It is the very adaptability that increases the risk of developing cancer. This may not seem obvious, so let me offer some further explanation.

When we are born, we simply have no idea which infections we shall encounter in our lives. Even common infections may mutate so that our immune system no longer recognises them. To encode in our genes the full set of immunological responses to counter every single possible infection would therefore be practically impossible. It would be like having to carry every single volume of the *Oxford English Dictionary* with you in case someone used a very rare word that you didn't understand. Instead we have evolved immunity, which can not only adapt but also store the memory of an encounter with an infection indefinitely.

For that to happen, the cells that store the memory of the encounter must alter their genes, permanently. They are then able to produce the necessary precise antibodies to combat the infection. This means that rearrangement of their genes has to occur. Further, to generate the huge range of possible antibody responses required, a state of 'hypermutation' has to arise. The rearrangement of genes associated with a state of hypermutation is almost identical to the basis of cancer, and is the principal mechanism by which our 'accelerator' is applied.

Infections are, therefore, mutagenic (ie, they induce mutations), in a very similar way to other more commonly thought-of causes of cancer such as radiation or chemicals. The example above applies very specifically to cells of immunity, in particular the variety of lymphocytes called B-cells, also known as memory cells for the reasons that must by now be obvious. Cancers of B-cells most definitely do occur, in a number of varieties. But how does this apply to, say, stomach or lung cancer? They are not required to generate an almost infinite variety of responses to infection in the way that B-cells are.

The connection between these types of cancer and our infection-induced hypermutability may seem less obvious. However, the signal that activates B-cells to begin the process of rearranging their genes is a chemical messenger called a cytokine. The effect of some cytokines is also to accelerate the growth of cells, and this function is not limited to particular cell types. This makes sense; if your tissues are infected, they will die and need to be replaced rapidly. It is the function of the cytokine to pass that information on to living cells. It is becoming clear that many cancers are stimulated by this mechanism, at the heart of which is long-term, chronic inflammation, usually as a result of infection. Certain cytokines almost certainly induce hypermutability and gene rearrangements in all cells. To be a living human, to survive inevitable encounters with infection, requires this trade-off, and that leads to a tendency to cancer. To meet the constant evolutionary challenge of infection we need to be permanently in a state of readiness to change; that change may be lethal to us.

I excluded one further infection that is associated with cancers from the brief list above, and that is the bacterium *Helicobacter pylori*. There is no doubt that this is a very common cancer-causing organism, which also causes stomach ulcers. The story of how this was discovered is a mixture of nobility, recklessness and genius that somehow seems to belong to an earlier stage of scientific exploration than our own.

Recklessness and genius

Barry Marshall is the son of a boilermaker, and was brought up in rural western Australia. His early life was spent in a house with a dirt floor and an outside toilet. The family had no car and no television. Life was hard, but Barry was bright and in 1969 managed to get in to the University of Western Australia. He originally planned to be an engineer, but changed his mind and began to study medicine. For much of his time at medical school he was a drifter, doing the bare minimum to get by. He very nearly chose the safer, less challenging career of becoming a family doctor, but ultimately ended up as a hospital physician, and looked for a research project to improve his prospects. As he himself said, he had been told at medical school that everything useful in medicine had already been discovered. That did not quite match with the reality of Marshall's own experience of numerous patients with untreatable conditions.

He was working at the Royal Perth Hospital when he ran into Robin Warren, a pathologist. Warren had a tendency to tell anyone who would listen that he kept seeing something odd down his microscope. In the biopsy specimens from patients with ulcers – which he had to scrutinise to make sure they had no cancerous cells – he was seeing tiny comma-shaped structures that seemed to resemble bacteria. Almost nobody would listen to Warren on this pet subject. Everyone 'knew' what caused ulcers: it was an excess of acid production, which could be treated with surgery or acid-blockers. It was also universally accepted that the potent acids of the stomach would annihilate and dissolve bacteria; there is no way they could live there. Marshall, though, had a quick and ready mind that was open to new ideas. He set about trying to grow the bacteria in the laboratory.

For months Marshall and Warren had no luck growing the bug. They tried different culture conditions, with different agar preparations, temperatures and atmospheres, but nothing seemed to work. It was one of those freak events that occur frequently in discovery that gave them their break. One Easter weekend the laboratory was closed for the holidays. Usually they inspected the Petri dishes after a couple of days, then threw them away because there was nothing growing. On this occasion, the holiday neglect had allowed the slow-growing organisms time to develop into visible colonies.

The excitement of this discovery was almost visceral to the ambitious Marshall. He was onto something big here, and he knew it. He also knew that his colleagues would be sceptical, and would dismiss his discovery as contamination of the plates. He knew he would struggle and probably fail to get permission to test his hypothesis on patients. So he decided to take radical action.

Marshall knew that he would have to prove to the world that his bacteria caused stomach ulcers; at some level he also needed to prove it to himself. Inoculating your infectious agent into a healthy victim, observing the symptoms and signs of the disease, and then recovering the infectious agent, provides virtually unassailable proof about the cause of an infectious disease. Marshall decided to test his hypothesis by swallowing a culture of his bacteria.

Sure enough, a week or so later he began to suffer the precise symptoms of ulcer disease. He was vomiting, had intense abdominal pain and clearly had gastritis. Marshall had convinced himself. Convincing the rest of the world was another matter. It took almost a decade before the hypothesis associating ulcers and the new bacterium was generally accepted, and the dogged persistence with which Marshall propagated his findings probably shortened the time even then.

Iconoclasts in medicine are not always immediately welcomed. One famous story which is often cited concerns Ignaz Semmel-weiss. He was a 19th-century Hungarian physician practising in

Vienna, who first advanced the theory that dangerous infections may be introduced into the birth canals of pregnant females by the hands of examining doctors, nurses and medical students. His observation was based upon the death of his friend and colleague Jakob Kolletschka, a pathologist who died of a condition very similar to the 'puerperal sepsis' he had seen kill so many pregnant mothers. Kolletschka had died after cutting his finger with a blade he was using for dissection, and Semmelweiss proposed that the cause of his death must be related to something he had acquired from the cadaver.

For his pains – suggesting that doctors might be the cause of a disease, rather than its cure – he was effectively rejected by the medical profession and ultimately died in a lunatic asylum. Some refer to the 'Semmelweiss reflex', which is a mule-headed reluctance to accept novel hypotheses. Semmelweiss lived some years before the 'germ' theory of disease was proven by Pasteur. His findings were largely rejected because they appeared at the time to have no scientific rationale. Ultimately, of course, he was vindicated but not before many thousands of women died unnecessarily from poor hand hygiene among medical staff.

The fact that patients are still dying from infections transmitted by medical staff who fail to wash their hands correctly suggests that the Semmelweiss reflex is alive and well. However, part of the problem was that Semmelweiss lacked Marshall's determination, and failed to publish his findings effectively in his own lifetime. The world of medicine was stood on its head by the *Helicobacter* story. Many countries, particularly in Asia, suffer gastric cancer in epidemic numbers. Marshall's breakthrough could help to prevent many such deaths.

Heart disease and infections

For a brief period it was believed that *Helicobacter pylori* was also a cause of heart disease. This turned out to be probably not true. The apparent association between the two reflected only the fact that both are associated with poverty. For the purposes of the theme of this book, it would have been satisfying to produce evidence of a convincing association between an infection and the West's biggest killer – heart disease – but that association would appear not to be with *Helicobacter*.

One of the great physicians, Sir William Osler, proposed a possible infectious link with heart attacks as long ago as 1908. Other infectious agents have been proposed – cytomegalovirus, for instance, and herpes. The most convincing to date has been a bacterium called *Chlamydia pneumoniae*. This is a relative of one of our other epidemic bacteria, *Chlamydia trachomatis*, the cause of an epidemic of sexually transmitted infections in the West.

C. pneumoniae has teetered on the brink of being proven a cause of heart disease for many years. Some studies seem to show an association between evidence of past infection with the bug and heart attacks, while others do not. Rabbits infected with the bacterium develop a condition very like ischaemic heart disease. The bug has been found in the plaques of fatty tissue in blood vessels that cause heart attacks. There is a convincing, rational hypothesis to explain the association. The infection could lead to local excessive production of inflammatory chemicals (the same cytokines involved in cancer), which are known to affect the way fats are handled in the body. The likelihood is that a multitude of factors – heredity, diet, lack of exercise – combine to cause furring of the arteries. The proven involvement of infection is indirect in that diabetes, itself a product of infection, predisposes people to heart attacks. Sadly for my purposes – and sadly for mankind, in that *C. pneumoniae* can be treated with antibiotics – the conclusive killer punch to prove the association with infection simply is not there. Yet.

Much of this chapter has dealt with associations with infection that are counter-intuitive, strange and far from obvious. They are as nothing, though, compared with the oddity of our next candidate, the one that has challenged our notions of living things and almost destroyed a way of life. This is the prion.

CHAPTER 8

PRIONS

BH was 56 years old. He had been deteriorating mentally for some years, and when I first met him he was effectively in a coma. He was being fed a liquid diet through a nasogastric tube, one that passes nutrients to the stomach through the nostril. His decline had been punctuated by moments of terror and paranoia, with trembling, poor coordination and ultimately loss of use of his limbs. We were asked to review him by our friends the neurologists; no cause for his decline had yet been found. Could he have Creutzfelt-Jacob disease, possibly the new variant supposedly transmitted from cows, known as vCJD? Some of the features of his illness fitted neatly. Terror and paranoia sometimes occur in vCJD. The progressive and relentless nature of his increasing disability was also suggestive, although the time course was a little longer than is usual.

The diagnosis of vCJD is an extremely difficult one to make, at least in life. Where some types of modern medical imaging (such as magnetic resonance imaging) may be suggestive, as may fluid from taken from around the brain, neither is conclusive. Sometimes tissue taken from the tonsils may yield the answer, but for absolute confirmation a biopsy of the brain is needed, or at least it was at the time we were asked to look at BH. This is a hazardous procedure in life. Often scarring in the brain can lead to disturbance of transmission of electrical impulses and epilepsy can result.

In this case we elected not to perform a brain biopsy. There was then absolutely no known treatment for vCJD; even now the treatments are unproven. The advantage in providing a diagnosis was at best marginal, and at worst the procedure would have left BH with fits in addition to his very severe loss of function. We made absolutely certain that no stone was left unturned in an effort to find any other cause for his condition – especially in case it was a treatable one, for instance syphilis – but felt that aggressive tests would be cruel and pointless.

BH died shortly afterwards, and at post-mortem we found that our judgement had been correct. He had suffered not from vCJD, but from a not dissimilar and also incurable condition called cerebral amyloid. I have never diagnosed a case of vCJD; this is not that surprising, as we shall discover. If bird flu is the Once and Future King of epidemics, then vCJD is the Great Pretender.

Mad cows and humans

The extraordinary story of bovine spongiform encephalopathy (BSE), or mad cow disease, has caused a rethink of one of the most basic tenets of biology. It has had catastrophic consequences for the livelihoods of many; in the form of vCJD it has also killed scores of human beings.

BSE was rapidly identified in cattle after it first appeared in the mid-1980s. Veterinary scientists have something of an advantage over medical doctors here; there is no ethical or moral dilemma in performing post-mortem examinations on slaughtered beef cattle. Obtaining consent for post-mortems in humans, especially where there are religious or cultural reasons that the corpse must be disposed of rapidly, can be awkward.

The veterinary scientists involved were presented with a relatively large number of specimens. They noticed that the brains of affected cows were 'spongy' in appearance, almost as though bubbles had appeared in the tissue, which was filled with tangled strands of protein-like tissue. They compared the appearances with other known diseases, and found the closest match was to a group of illnesses in humans and animals caused by what were then known as slow viruses. Nobody had actually ever identified these viruses, but in the absence of any identifiable bacterium, fungus or parasite it was assumed that there must be a viral cause. The diseases in animals were scrapie in sheep, mink encephalopathy, and chronic wasting disease in deer. The pattern in humans resembled *kuru* (which means 'trembling disease'), a disease encountered principally among tribes in New Guinea who practised cannibalism, and a number of hereditary conditions including Creutzfeldt-Jakob and Gerstmann Straussler disease.

The feature that these illnesses had in common was the appearance of the tangled mats of protein in the brain. There seemed to be two means of acquiring the disease, either heredity or exposure to the right (or wrong) sort of tissue. Thus *kuru* only seemed to occur in cannibals. Creutzfeldt-Jakob, in its acquired form, was found in people who had received transplanted human tissue, more particularly derived from the brain. For some years children who were deficient in growth hormone were given extracts from human pituitary glands in an attempt to make them grow taller. Some of these children developed CJD, the so-called iatrogenic form.

Not unreasonably the concern was raised that the agent of disease – the slow virus – might transfer to humans from infected cattle. Previously scientists had been reassured that sheep had suffered the similar disease of scrapie for many generations, and the disease had not passed to people. However, the fact that the illness was occurring in a new species sounded a warning to alert scientists. Once a disease can leap one species barrier, there is absolutely no reason that it should not leap another.

'If bovine spongiform encephalopathy turns out to be infectious, it could cause problems out of proportion to the number of cases.' These words come from the *New Scientist*'s news service, posted on the internet on 5 November 1987. Given the disastrous outcome of the virtual annihilation of the British beef industry, could there have been more prophetic words than these?

Those alarm bells seemed timely. A new disease appeared to be emerging, similar to the hereditary variant of CJD but with two cruel twists. The age range of the people afflicted was far younger, and the illness progressed much more rapidly. The first victim died of the new disease in May 1995, one of three that year. The following year there were ten victims, then another ten, then 18.

The epidemic that changed epidemics

Prions are the epidemic that changed epidemics. The central dogma of biology until prions were described was that all living and infectious tissue relied upon nucleic acids – genetic material – for its own reproduction. In other words, every single infectious agent that had ever been described, since the 'germ' theory of disease was proven by Pasteur, turned out to contain genes. Except prions.

The suggestion that the transmissible spongiform encephalopathies (TSEs) might be something other than conventional infectious material has been around since the 1960s, long before the term 'prion' was coined. This theory arose from two key observations, made by radiation biologist Tikvah Alper and physicist J S Griffith. The first was that the 'slow virus' believed to cause scrapie and Creutzfeldt-Jakob disease seemed impervious to ultra-violet radiation. That should not happen. The nucleic acids of viruses are supposed to be destroyed easily by UV light. However, these 'slow viruses' were destroyed by agents that disrupted proteins. This was a fascinating insight, but one with only academic interest until the advent of mad cow disease, when it suddenly became very important indeed.

Stanley B Prusiner of the University of California, San Francisco led the team which confirmed that the infectious agent consisted of a single protein. In 1982 Prusiner coined the word 'prion' as a name for the infectious agent, by combining the first two syllables of the words 'proteinaceous' and 'infectious'. This research won Prusiner the Nobel Prize for Medicine in 1997.

What then is a prion, and how does it work? What are they for? Suppose you are a bricklayer, building a house. The stability of the wall you build relies on the regularity and stability of the bricks you receive from the brickworks. Now suppose there is a problem with the brickmaking process, such that one of every few bricks is made of defective material. Superficially these bricks appear normal, and you do not notice anything odd about them as you create your perfect, regular structure. However, when you visit the site a few weeks later, the architect points out to you that some of the bricks have started to twist and deform, to crack the neighbouring bricks, and to disrupt the beautiful wall you had worked so carefully to create. The whole edifice is now unstable.

Prions work by affecting the 'bending' of adjacent proteins, just like the twisting housebricks that damage their neighbours. Those proteins become functionally abnormal, and are laid down in tangled, matted fibrils. This occurs particularly in nervous tissue. That does not really answer the question of what they are actually for. Why did the brickmaker deliver twisting bricks? There is a continuing debate about whether prions in fungi and plants are useful agents employed by species for their own ends, or whether they represent disease, as they do in humans.

The evidence for the useful functions of prions is patchy, but there is some. Of the actions that have been suggested, one is that they may be responsible for the permanent imprinting of memory in the brain. Prions are resistant to the natural means of breaking down redundant proteins, the enzymes called proteases, and it can be seen that this might be useful if permanence is a necessary property. Mice that are incapable of making prions have defects in the hippocampus, part of the brain vital for memory processing. In our brickmaking analogy, it might be that the factory needed to use flexible, twisting (and indestructible) bricks to record a template, or memory, for the design of new types, and that some of these were delivered in error. In the chapter on fungi, I briefly outlined their action in restricting the access of rival fungal species to a cooperative colony (see pages 161–62). Here perhaps, to follow our house analogy, the brickmaker might have accidentally sent the sort of brick he used as flexible spacers between pallets.

The epidemic that wasn't

Why did I call vCJD the Great Pretender? To produce prion disease, the individual must have a hereditary susceptibility. This was the basis of the predictions for the ultimate mortality of vCJD, in that the evidence suggested that enormous numbers of us carry the genes that make us theoretically at risk. Not every house is made of bricks; those made of other materials might be immune to the dangerous brickmaker. The initial prediction for the potential mortality of vCJD in the UK, based on the frequency of the gene for susceptibility in the general population, was 10 million.

All the cases so far have occurred in people with particular versions of genes related to the prion protein that is the key to the disease. These people make up 40 per cent of the population. In 2002, the prediction dropped to 50,000, based on data up to

the year 2000. In 2003 the figure was revised to a range somewhere between 7,000 and 10. In reality the number of deaths
between 2003 and the end of 2006 (the most recent available
data) has been 37, about 12 per year, in a trend which continues
to decline. The prediction in 2003 was for 30 deaths in
2004/2005 (the actual number was 14). The peak year was 2000,
when there were 28 deaths. Even supposing we were to return to
that peak (not an unreasonable prediction, given the supposed
incubation period of vCJD), we would still struggle to meet the
projected number of 7,000 deaths by 2070, let alone 10 million.

Has there ever been another disease in human history where
the gap between prediction and reality has been so prodigious?
To be fair, the group that drew up these figures only looked at
cases and deaths from people thought to have become infected
with vCJD by eating infected meat. Their study does not
include secondary transmission of the illness, which could theoretically occur from human to human via infected surgical
instruments or blood transfusions.

It should also be noted that prions are astonishingly robust.
We have noted that they are not destroyed by ultra-violet light,
or protein-destroying protease enzymes. Nor are they destroyed
by chemical disinfection or extremes of heat, possibly including
incineration, giving rise to the possibility that billions of prion
particles might have been released into the soil by burning cattle
carcases, and we have not seen the last of this disease.

If the presumption that prions serve useful biological functions is correct, then we find ourselves back with the basic
premise of this book. Humans are susceptible to prion diseases
because of their own essential structure. This is more than

simply saying that prion diseases can only occur in the susceptible, because of the existence of both the hereditary and
transmissible forms. There are no other (known) diseases that
occur like this. Infectious diseases may be acquired or congeni-
tal – present at birth, like syphilis. However, syphilis is not
encoded in the genes of sufferers, and has to be acquired by the
mother before it can transmit to the baby. There are hereditary
diseases, present at birth, like cystic fibrosis, but it is not infectious. Prions are implicated in the only diseases capable of both
states, both genetically acquired and transmissible.

Just desserts?

Given the consistent theme of this book, it would be easy to
construct an argument along the lines that diseases like BSE and
vCJD are the inevitable consequence of humans interfering
with natural processes. Cows have not evolved to eat other
cows, or the products of other animals. Cows have evolved as
ruminants, which digest vegetable matter, and should be
permitted to remain as such. It can hardly be surprising that a
disease once confined to cannibals should rear its head when
cows are forced into cannibalism. This, of all the epidemics we
have discussed, seems the most conspicuously of our own
creation.

This line of reasoning does partly support the main premise of
this book. However, it is not a line of argument that I endorse. It
implies that there is something immoral about interfering with
nature, and that we obtain our just desserts when nature delivers
us something like BSE and vCJD in revenge.

There are a number of essential flaws in this argument. One is the fact that it is speculative anyway, as the case for vCJD being caused by a prion remains unproven. Recently a team led by Yale University neuropathologist Laura Manuelidis claimed to have discovered a virus responsible for the TSEs. Nevertheless the conventional view remains that it is the prion that lies at the heart of the disease.

More tellingly, I would contend that it is impossible to specify convincingly what is 'natural' in our world. Clean water; central heating; antibiotics; electric light; dentistry; agriculture (even organic and free range); pain-killing drugs: none is truly 'natural' in the sense that they are free from the artifice of humans. It is by manipulating 'nature', through our ever more sophisticated use of tools, that the human animal defines itself. It does not matter whether that tool is a flint knife, a machine for rendering cow carcases into cattle feed, or a computer that generates wildly inaccurate predictions about the ultimate mortality of an outbreak. We became victim to the vCJD outbreak not because we offended nature, but because such things are in our nature. We would probably not make the same mistake again, but on purely practical principles rather than because of our fretting over sins against nature.

I would make a further point about the catastrophic consequences of this minor if peculiarly unpleasant epidemic. Many hundreds of thousands of cattle were slaughtered on the basis that vCJD was probably being transmitted to humans. It is one of the central principles of our understanding of the modern western epidemic of heart disease and obesity that an excess of dietary fats is in part responsible. There is also convincing evidence that an excess of dietary red meat may contribute to colonic cancer. We cannot blame the government of Britain and the European Union of the time for taking the action that they did, based on the evidence of its experts, and it is likely that further cases of vCJD were prevented by the radical measures adopted, Nevertheless one cannot help asking what the overriding principle of the government's health policy must be, if it takes action to prevent vCJD from spreading, but takes no action to stop us all eating red meat to prevent colonic cancer.

The difference between vCJD and mortality through eating red meat is the acceptability in political terms of tackling one versus the other. The mortality from heart disease massively dwarfs vCJD, as does that from colonic cancer. The latter accounts for 56,000 deaths in the United States, 17,000 in the United Kingdom, with a million new cases worldwide per year. Of course, the government was planning its strategy based on expert advice that 10 million might be at risk of vCJD.

Prion diseases are unfortunately untreatable, although the drugs quinacrine and pentosan polyphosphate have been tried. This leads us neatly to our next chapter, which is the epidemic of diseases that have become untreatable. We shall now talk about resistance.

CHAPTER 9

RESISTANCE!

The resistance of epidemics to antimicrobial drugs is unquestionably an emerging threat. In this regard it is the one that can most easily be said to be human-made. This is the epidemic that we have brought upon ourselves. In fact, as was made clear in other chapters, our behaviour has brought about many of the outbreaks of infectious disease that have swept our planet over the millennia. Naked commercial greed brought diseases with disastrous consequences both to and from the New World. The Old World exported measles and smallpox, and got yellow fever and (possibly) syphilis in return. Changes in sexual behaviour, plus poverty and global economic migration, have permitted the great scourge of modern times – HIV/AIDS – to emerge with catastrophic consequences. Complacency about the threat from tuberculosis certainly helped bring about the outbreak in New York in the early 1990s.

In terms of actual numbers, the threat from resistance

remains relatively small, when compared with the overall figures for infectious disease, and the problem has until recently been confined to hospitals rather than widespread in the community. This is of little comfort if you happen to become infected with a resistant organism. Furthermore it is a situation that shows every likelihood of becoming worse, not better. According to the US National Institute of Allergy and Infectious Diseases, 2 million patients will acquire an infection during their stay in hospital each year. Of these, 90,000 will die, a figure up from 13,300 in 1992. Of those infections, 70 per cent demonstrate resistance to at least one antibiotic, making such infections harder to treat, and requiring more expensive and more toxic drugs. The same is true, to a point, with malaria, which in some parts of the world has become resistant to several of the commonly used drugs. Some believe that resistance to the newer drugs, and to older, more toxic ones like quinine, will emerge eventually. This is an epidemic that is gathering strength.

Nick's story

Nick was a heroin addict aged 35. He had been 'shooting up' intermittently since he was 18. Nick was well educated and intelligent, his background being almost aristocratic. In the earlier years of his addiction he had held a stable job and had been able to afford drugs of good quality. He had kept his 'works' – the paraphernalia of syringes and needles required to maintain his habit – in good order. In later years, though, in a fairly common pattern, his life had declined, he had lost his job and his standards had fallen. The veins in his arms had collapsed and scarred up through regular stabbing to get his daily fix. He now had to resort to injecting into the major blood vessel that runs through the groin, the femoral vein. Further evidence for his plight was blatant to us: his blood tests revealed that he had both hepatitis B and hepatitis C, doubtless acquired from contaminated needles. He was lucky in that so far he had escaped HIV. However, his luck was about to run out.

He came to our hospital as an emergency admission with a fever, fatigue, sweats and breathlessness which had been developing over the previous week. By the time I attended the Emergency Department the diagnosis was effectively made. Simply by observing his chest X-ray I could see the classic evidence of abscesses in his lungs. There could be no real doubt what was wrong. Careful listening to his chest through a stethoscope revealed the characteristic hiss of turbulent blood flow through his heart valves. The source was easily revealed when I examined the injection site in his groin. There was a moderate-sized abscess forming a tented lump in the centre of a patch of angry red inflammation. Nick had endocarditis. He had transferred the bacteria from his abscess into his bloodstream. They had settled on his heart valve, which was already damaged by the constant stream of talcum powder and other contaminants with which his heroin had been cut by unscrupulous dealers.

Over the following days we had to amend Nick's antibiotics to counter the organism that was growing all too readily from his blood and from his abscess. The bacterium was MRSA. This was a grave problem. Although there are antibiotics that are active against the resistant variant of *Staphylococcus aureus*, they are simply not as lethal to bacteria as drugs like penicillin, as well as being more toxic. We strove to optimise his dose, and gave him the best available treatment. Nick had been in and out of various hospitals with various problems. It was difficult to be certain whether he had acquired his MRSA from one of those visits, or had caught it in the community, where the bacterium is increasingly common.

Matters progressed badly for Nick. He began to develop tiny black streaks under his fingernails and angry blotches in the blood vessels under his eyelids. An ultrasound test of his heart confirmed what we suspected – the infection had spread from the tricuspid valve in the right side of his heart to the aortic valve on the left. This is far more dangerous, because the bacteria now had access to all of his tissues, as the left chambers of the heart pump blood to all parts of the body, not just the lungs. Worryingly, his kidneys were beginning to struggle.

Rapid progression of endocarditis of this nature demands urgent surgery to remove the damaged and infected tissue. If the main heart valve ruptures from infection, the strain on the heart is simply too great and the pump fails. In desperation we transferred him to intensive care and urgently called our surgical colleagues. Sadly, though, Nick abruptly deteriorated and died. At post-mortem it was found that an abscess had formed around the base of his aorta (the main blood vessel), which had burst.

One of the tragedies among the many illustrated by this story is that Nick would probably have survived had he infected himself with a strain of bacteria that was sensitive to penicillin or one of its cousins. However, MRSA is becoming increasingly common worldwide, both in hospital practice and in the community. How did this come to be? To understand that, we need to return to the very origins of the widespread availability of effective antibiotics.

The antibiotic problem

Most people will be aware that resistance arises through the indiscriminate prescribing of antibiotics. That, though, is only half the story. The other half is the remarkable capacity of microorganisms to generate mechanisms for resistance. Compared with higher organisms, bacteria have relatively few genes. Thus small mutations will have profound consequences for the function of the organism. But there is more.

Let us go back to the proverbial beginning. The account of Fleming's initial observation of penicillin is so widely known as to be almost folklore. It is worth recalling a single fact about the mould that drifted from the pub opposite through his laboratory window at St Mary's Hospital in London, and from there into his Petri dish. That fact is that the mould was a naturally occurring creature, and that the penicillin it exuded was its natural product. Within a very short period Fleming was able to observe that some colonies of bacteria, initially susceptible to the substance produced by *Penicillium*, lost their susceptibility. The fact that these bacteria were able to acquire this property so rapidly tells us something crucial about the way that such organisms treat our attempts to destroy them. It is with contempt, in fact.

In the natural world microorganisms do not live in isolation. They compete for territory and food in exactly the way that higher organisms do. In doing so, sometimes they need to fend off or even kill rivals. At the microscopic level of the causes of epidemics, the weapons used are not horns, claws and teeth, but chemicals like penicillin. Precisely as other life-forms evolve defensive mechanisms, so bacteria have evolved antidotes to fungal penicillin. The staphylococci that Fleming observed were doing exactly this, pumping out an enzyme that inactivates penicillin called beta-lactamase.

We have previously mentioned that, until very recently, almost all antibiotics were derived from natural sources such as fungi in sewage outfalls. Putting all of this together, you should be able to see immediately where this argument is going. Bacteria have no difficulty in producing 'antidotes' to these poisons, and the development of resistance to such compounds is less a likelihood than an inevitability.

This is a ready explanation of how bacteria can develop resistance to antibiotics derived from fungi. Scientists have moved on, though, and newer antibiotics have been developed that are entirely synthetic and unlike anything in the 'natural' world. It might be predicted that bacteria would struggle to engineer mechanisms to counter them. Indeed, some antibacterials were announced with a fanfare on precisely this premise. Linezolid is an example. It is a drug initially developed in 1987 for the treatment of MRSA (among other infections), and it was widely believed that resistance to it would never emerge. It was one of the drugs we tried to use for poor Nick. It was licensed in the United States in 2000. The first Linezolid-resistant strain of MRSA emerged in Britain in 2001 and in America in 2003.

As Dr David Livermore, director of the Britain's Health Protection Agency Antimicrobial Resistance Monitoring and Reference Laboratory, said at the time, 'We must not lose sight of the fact that antibiotic-resistance is a demonstration of evolution – the life force of nature. As we use antibiotics we inevitably select for resistance – all that varies is the time scale.' Bacteria thus treat any synthetic chemical in exactly the same way as they do penicillin. It simply takes them a little longer to figure out a way to defeat it. In doing this the bacteria simply obey the same principles that all life-forms do.

This property brings bacteria closer to some aspects of human evolution. In order for them to develop Linezolid resistance, adaptations must emerge that are different from the susceptible, wild strain. In the case of Linezolid, this means that they must find a different way of synthesising proteins, because that is where the drug acts against them. As a general rule, such adapted bacteria are less 'fit' than their wild cousins. Exposure to Linezolid kills all the fitter, susceptible organisms, and those mutants that have a 'defective' means of protein synthesis can occupy the vacant niche. In time further adaptations may make the new strain fitter again, but the principle is identical to one we have met in humans. It is the same as balanced polymorphism, where disadvantageous genes such as sickle-cell or cystic fibrosis persist because of our exposure to malaria and tuberculosis. Thus we and epidemics are alike, because we are obliged to obey the same evolutionary mechanisms, David Livermore's 'life force of nature'.

We can add to this knowledge another skill of bacteria, and that is the capacity to share information. This takes many forms, but one method is via chunks of their own genes. These are called mobile genetic elements, and they have profound implications for human as well as bacterial evolution. They are discussed in Chapters 3 and 10. As far as bacteria are concerned, they are a means whereby genes encoding resistance can be transferred both among and between species. Some bacteria are especially skilled at this, and once resistance is established it can spread like wildfire among communities and hospitals.

The resisters

MRSA is far from the only bacterium in which resistance has developed. *Klebsiella, Pseudomonas, Acinetobacter, Burkholderia*: strains of each have become highly resistant to just about every antibiotic in the pharmacy, and kill as a consequence. The majority have done so within the hospital environment. Unlike MRSA they usually kill only the very sick. The method by which each has developed its skill is serial exposure to the various antibiotics, coupled with a capacity for sharing genetic material.

However, this is not the only means by which resistance has emerged. Antibiotics used as growth promoters in agriculture – avoparcin is the most widely quoted – have permitted widespread resistance to emerge. The most troublesome of the organisms that has resulted is the Vancomycin-resistant enterococcus (VRE). What is fascinating about this particular bacterium is that resistance arose in different species of animals, and the subsequent spread into humans can be plotted by variations in the mutant genes. Thus people who eat no pork but only chicken get chicken VRE, and vice versa. Tens of thousands of kilos of avoparcin have entered the food chain via agriculture. In some senses we live in a dilute solution of antibiotics. We live with the consequences of our own cleverness.

Resistance!

It is not only bacteria and protozoa that can develop resistance. Neil was possibly one of the best-educated patients I have ever encountered. He had degrees from several first-rate British universities, played several musical instruments at concert level, spoke numerous languages and sang in a cathedral choir. He had contracted HIV relatively early in the epidemic. His intelligence and wide reading had meant that he had kept up with every advance in medication for his condition. His company was both stimulating and taxing; we all knew that we had better be on our toes and have read the latest research before a consultation with him. He was articulate and forceful enough to have successfully requested each new drug as it became available. This was to be his undoing.

Drugs for the HIV epidemic became available one after the other. The very first was AZT, also known as zidovudine, which had previously failed as a drug for cancer in 1964. It was licensed for treatment of HIV in 1987. Others followed – didanosine in 1991, stavudine in 1994, saquinavir in 1995. It was not until 1996 that it became clear that a combination of drugs was needed to suppress the virus reliably. Until that point patients given each agent in series demonstrated some suppression of the virus followed by a resurgence. The reason for this was depressingly reliable – resistance. The virus simply found ways of permanently evading the action of the drugs. So this had happened to Neil. By the time I met him he had acquired resistance to every known class of HIV drug. He finally died of cancer related to the AIDS we had been unable to suppress, a tragic loss of a supremely able and intelligent young man.

The paradox of HIV/AIDS is that what allowed us to attack it now risks stealing the advantage away from us in the form of resistance. This is because of the nature of the virus itself. HIV belongs to a group of viruses called retroviruses, or lentiviruses. They have a number of key properties, the first of which is that the genes of the virus are made of RNA. In order for the virus to achieve its aims of incorporating into the DNA-based genes of the host, this needs to be converted into DNA. The two types of gene are incompatible; RNA cannot incorporate into DNA, and vice versa.

Retroviruses are unusual in that they carry the mechanism for converting RNA to DNA, in the form of a pre-made enzyme called reverse transcriptase. This enzyme is, by the standards of mammalian enzymes, sloppy and of poor quality. By this I mean that it is very poor at proof-reading, at checking its own error rate, and in deciding what to incorporate in the growing chain of DNA formed from its own template. Drugs like AZT make use of this property. AZT resembles the building blocks of DNA but with a key difference: it cannot bind the next block of the chain, and thus DNA transcription is terminated. Much choosier human enzymes generally ignore AZT when synthesising new DNA chains, and are thus broadly spared its effects.

It is also the sloppiness of HIV reverse transcriptase that allows resistance to develop. Viruses that rely on such enzymes have a high rate of spontaneous mutation. An infected person may produce from 10 billion to 1,000 billion new viral particles per day. Inevitably some of these will be mutants, because reverse transcriptase is so careless. Exactly like our bacterial mutants, in the 'wild' untreated state these viral mutants will be less fit, and will die without progeny. This abruptly changes when drugs are introduced into the equation. The mutant that is capable of ignoring drugs like AZT, or even of using them, will be at a survival advantage and will thus emerge. If the drug is withdrawn, the resistant mutant may appear to vanish, but it will reappear if the drug is reinstated.

Despite the advent of combination therapy for HIV, known as 'highly active antiretroviral therapy', resistance still emerges. There are many reasons for this: people find the drugs hard to take, forget them, run out, are not properly supervised, develop intolerable side-effects, and a host of others. Resistance is most reliably evoked by partial exposure of the virus to the drug. Consistent and reliable treatment seems to suppress the virus adequately to prevent it developing. Ensuring this happens is a gruelling task involving close cooperation between doctor, nurse and patient, as well as expensive back-up laboratory facilities. I emphasise this for reasons that will become clear below.

We now know that a resistant virus may be transmitted from person to person. This may seem obvious, but for some time it was believed that the fitness disadvantage of a mutant virus might prevent that happening. Resistant strains of virus are now far from rare. Although the figure is falling, in 2003 nearly 11 per cent of people throughout Europe with new infections had evidence of resistance. In the United Kingdom the figure rose to 27 per cent at one time, although lately it appears to have fallen to levels closer to the rest of Europe.

These figures are from wealthy European countries. Careful supervision of the sort provided by advanced healthcare in such nations is crucial for controlling resistance. Experience from the treatment of tuberculosis in poorer nations warns us of the dangers of chaotic management of infectious disease. In Kazakhstan between 1999 and 2002, for instance, 57 per cent of *Mycobacterium tuberculosis* was resistant to at least one drug. A more extreme situation may arise where the bacterium becomes resistant to multiple drugs (MDR-TB), and becomes almost untreatable, as happened to Gaynor in Chapter 2. This has already begun to happen in some parts of the world. In Kazakhstan, Israel, Tomsk Oblast in Russia, Karakalpakstan in Uzbekistan, Estonia, the Lianoning and Henan provinces of China, and Lithuania, the prevalence of MDR-TB approaches 8 per cent. Tuberculosis, like HIV, is no respecter of national boundaries. There is absolutely no reason that epidemics of resistant disease from both causes should not be transmitted to neighbouring countries and worldwide. This is an epidemic that is coming to a hospital near you.

Here is the point: human interference with epidemics of infectious disease must be carried out with complete rigour and perseverance. Otherwise a further, secondary epidemic of the same illness will follow, only with the disastrous rider that it has become untreatable. The TB experience has provided us with a clear warning, with a conclusion that is contrary to popular, received opinion. There has been much pressure from some quarters to provide cheap or even free medication for poorer nations, and to permit the manufacture of 'generic' drugs that are active against HIV, free from restrictive patent. This is worthy enough, but it could be argued that without the expensive health services required to supervise treatment, and ensure it is rigorous enough to prevent resistance developing, there is potential for catastrophe here. Many of the countries with the highest prevalence and mortality from HIV/AIDS, predictably have the least effective healthcare systems. Of course we should not draw the conclusion that poor countries with rudimentary health care should be denied antiretroviral treatment. The point I am making is that cheap drugs are only a part of a very much more complex problem.

Our scientific understanding of the capacity for bacteria and viruses to evade successive agents that are directed against them suggests a further more troubling possibility. Science is not always directed for benign purposes. In recent years it has become possible to extract genes for properties such as antibiotic resistance from bacteria and viruses, and splice them into another organism to produce an artificial, hybrid product. This might be, for example, smallpox with a gene for resistance to the vaccine, or a common and transmissible agent like the common cold which is inherently very different to treat, with a more toxic property spliced into it. Such manipulation of viruses is easily within the scope of many laboratories in the world. There is no reason that such a hybrid virus could not be released by some organisation with the skill and the motivation to carry out this kind of biowarfare.

I shall end this chapter with the slightly more hopeful suggestion that resistance may operate in more than one direction. Humans can demonstrate resistance to the most lethal and relentless of infections. In Chapter 1, we discussed the CCR5 delta-32 mutation, which confers resistance to HIV. We have encountered other examples of the phenomenon of balanced polymorphism, where we trade off hereditary illness against susceptibility to infectious diseases like tuberculosis. Once again, this simply reflects our kinship with the agents of infection. We obey the same rules of life, and resistance to disease emerges among us too.

CHAPTER 10

'NEW' EPIDEMICS

Cunning, innovative, inventive, inquisitive and rapacious: those human qualities, which have served us so well in improving our lot, are exactly the same ones that are getting us into trouble now with new infectious diseases. The quiddity of being a human takes us to new habitats (usually to exploit and destroy them), and places us and our livestock where we do not 'belong'. In terms of new infectious epidemics, this is the source of the coming threats. We know this from the past and from the present. Each of the major new epidemics of the 20th and early 21st centuries has arisen from this route, and the same was true in earlier centuries.

Consider yellow fever, the unpleasant mosquito-borne viral illness which killed tens of thousands in the Americas and Europe from the 17th to early 20th centuries. The craving of humans for sugar meant mass deforestation of Caribbean islands in order to plant cane. Birds and monkeys lost their habitat, and the mosquitoes that fed from them were forced to find new hosts. They found them in the shape of the slaves and settlers who were clearing the land. The mosquitoes carried the monkey disease with them. Many people died, and others were shipped around the world as part of the slave trade to infect cities as far away as Barcelona and Pittsburgh.

It remains to be seen whether climate change will cause old epidemics to trouble us in new places. There is convincing evidence that existing diseases such as malaria and Dengue fever are changing their distribution because of higher global temperatures. This is most pronounced in higher altitudes, because temperature changes are exaggerated there. We have seen malaria spreading ever higher in the Andes, and in some African nations. Coupled with emerging malarial resistance this could be said to be a new epidemic.

Richard's story

Richard was 22, and had been travelling on a gap year after finishing university. He was in Indonesia when the 2004 Boxing Day tsunami struck. He was lucky – he was inland when the surge of water carried away so many tourists and locals. He elected to stay on for a while to help with the rescue effort. His father was a friend of one of my colleagues. He rang us and asked us to see his son, who had become unwell with a headache. Richard was reluctant to come. He said he simply had sunburn, and wanted to stay at home to come to terms with the horrors he had witnessed.

When he arrived at our hospital you could indeed have been forgiven for thinking that he had spent too long in the sun. His face was pink and angry-looking. He was also somewhat withdrawn and morose, understandably, and had something of a headache. When we persuaded him to undress it became clear that there was more to this than just exposure to the sun's glare. The redness of his skin was not confined to those areas we might have expected. It extended over his entire body, and he also had some swollen lymph nodes in his neck and groin. A simple blood test revealed he was deficient in white blood cells, particularly the platelets which help the blood to clot, and also showed that he had no malaria parasites. We made a provisional diagnosis of Dengue; it was confirmed a few days later when his blood tested positive for the virus in the local reference laboratory.

Richard was lucky. A proportion of sufferers develop a haemorrhagic variety of Dengue, where the blood fails to clot. This can be fatal. Mass cases of Dengue were predicted after the tsunami. The disease, spread by the same mosquito that transmits yellow fever, is endemic in the countries the tsunami affected. Fortunately the epidemic never materialised, although it is not clear whether that was through chance or because of public health measures.

What is clear, though, is that the distribution of Dengue is changing, almost certainly as a consequence of global warming. Like malaria, the disease and its mosquito are appearing at ever higher altitudes. In the Columbian Andes, *Aedes aegypti* mosquitoes, which can carry the Dengue and yellow fever viruses, were previously limited to 3,300 ft (1,000 m) but now appear at 7,200 ft (2,200 m). In Mexico Dengue fever has spread above its former elevation limit of 3,300 ft (1,000 m) and has appeared at 5,600 ft (1,700 m).

Zoonoses

Dengue is an exception, because it does not fit the pattern of new epidemics in that it only appears to affect humans. Malaria does affect animals, but the parasites are different and cannot infect us. It is the close approximation of man to wild and peridomestic animals that has brought about the major recent threats. These are the zoonoses, and they form a very long list. The most prominent recent culprits have been severe acute respiratory syndrome (SARS), West Nile fever, HIV/AIDS and avian influenza. Many other illnesses of infection have arisen from the same source, and some even believe that the major infectious killer of the 19th century – *Mycobacterium tuberculosis* – is a mutated form of *Mycobacterium bovis*, the cattle variant. In fact examination of the genes of the two organisms suggests that it probably happened the other way around.

The source of some zoonoses has been exotic and bizarre. SARS almost certainly arose from Chinese culinary delicacies such as Tiger-Phoenix-Dragon soup. In this dish the tiger is the civet cat, the phoenix the chicken, and the dragon the cobra. Civet cats are actually species of mongoose. Such animals harbour many diseases, viral, bacterial and parasitic. As a general rule humans do not contract them unless contact is intimate. Mosquitoes, biting flies, lice and ticks form one such route, where mingling of blood in the bite avoids the natural defence of skin, but eating and butchery is another. In the winter of 2002–03 SARS arose in the Guangdong province of China, where civet cats are commonly butchered and eaten. Many of the initial victims were restaurant workers, and when the virus was identified it was found to be very closely related to a virus found in the intestine of civets.

The disease began to attract international attention later in 2003, when cases began to appear in Hong Kong. Between February 2003 and July 2003 there were 8,098 cases from 29 countries, including Canada, Taiwan and Singapore. There were 774 deaths, giving the disease a mortality of around 10 per cent. One of the earliest deaths was a Chinese doctor visiting Hong Kong. Subsequent mapping of the outbreak revealed that most of the early victims had stayed in the same hotel, although none seemed to have had close contact with the doctor.

Ultimately it was found that all of the victims had either passed through China or nursed earlier victims. The disease died out (for now) through good luck and global public health measures such as thermal imaging to detect people with fever passing through airports. The illness was characterised by high fever and difficulty in breathing, to the point of needing artificial ventilation, and even death. There is no proven effective treatment.

I never saw a case of SARS, although I was working in a department to which suspected cases were referred. In Britain this amounted to tiny numbers, certainly fewer than 20; as I recall it might have been six. There are those who believe that global warming, or at least warm weather, saved Europe from a mass epidemic. That spring was exceptionally warm, sunny and dry. Coronaviruses like SARS transmit by relatively close contact, or through inanimate objects like lift buttons. In that spring most of us were outdoors enjoying the sunshine. This made it far harder to transmit the virus in the numbers required for a true epidemic to establish itself. This is speculative, but it does carry the implication that next time we may not be so lucky.

The pattern of 'new' epidemics

We have not been lucky with some of the other 'new' epidemics that are troubling us now, and which follow the pattern of humans interfering with exotic environments. West Nile fever is now firmly established in many parts of the world including Europe and America. It arrived in New York in 1999, and has now affected every US state except Hawaii. It is not a new virus in the sense that it was first described in Uganda in the 1930s, but it had never previously been diagnosed in the West. It is believed to have arrived at New York Zoo with imported birds, and spread to local wild birds, especially crows. There were 3,000 cases in 2005, with 118 deaths in that year alone.

This has been a disturbing prelude to other bird-borne viruses. Unlike influenza the disease requires the additional agent of a mosquito to infect humans and horses. Unlike, say, malaria or yellow fever it is not at all choosy about the species of mosquito. There has not yet been a proven case of West Nile in Britain, although we have looked hard enough for cases. It is a nasty condition involving fever and meningitis, sometimes causing fatal encephalitis. If I wanted to find cases I would not have to travel far – they have been found in France, our nearest European neighbour.

This has been the pattern of 'new' infections to date. Nipah and Hendra viruses arose in fruit bats and were transmitted to humans, pigs and horses, the former in pig farmers in Malaysia and the latter in horses and their carers in Australia. Rather like West Nile, both cause an unpleasant, sometimes fatal encephalitis.

It should be obvious now where the modern threats are emerging. With the qualified exception of resistant bacteria, the principal source is our contact with animals. Of the 18 infectious diseases listed by the US National Institute of Allergy and Infectious Diseases as emerging threats, only tuberculosis, smallpox and group A Streptococcal infections have no involvement with animals. Antimicrobial resistance is clearly classified as an emerging threat; as we saw earlier, there is a clear connection with animals where antibiotics like avoparcin have been used in enormous quantities as agricultural growth promoters.

At the time of writing avian influenza remains a zoonosis, as its name suggests. As was explained in Chapter 1, the organism is incapable of binding to human tissues except following very intimate contact of the sort obtained by butchering or in industrial poultry houses. Thus the strain affecting birds cannot be transmitted reliably between humans. Were the virus to mutate only slightly, the situation might change radically to our disadvantage.

Avian influenza differs from the other zoonoses in that it has not really been mass human incursion into alien habitats that has caused it to emerge, or at least threaten to do so (unless you, not unreasonably, consider industrial poultry houses an alien environment). However, the great influenza pandemic of the early 20th century was certainly amplified by human folly and stupidity. It followed demobilised troops returning home in their millions at the end of the First World War, the war to end all wars, the Great War.

Where HIV might have come from

Nowhere are the consequences of the curiosity and rapacity of humans better illustrated than in the (hypothesised) origins of HIV. This illness appeared in significant numbers in the early 1980s. As it became clear which groups were at risk – homosexual men, intravenous drug users, ethnic minorities – all kinds of feverish and paranoid speculation broke out. Some said it was a right-wing plot to rid the United States of unwanted social groups. Others believed it had come from outer space on a meteorite. There was a theory promulgated by Edward Hooper in his book *The River*, that polio vaccine had become contaminated with a monkey virus which had mutated to affect humans. It briefly acquired credibility until rigorous scientific analysis disproved it. In reality the most likely origins of the disease are more bizarre than any of these.

Viruses contain clocks. This may seem an odd statement, but it is a crucial one for deciding how and when they appear. The clock is not, of course, an actual one, but a deductive, analogous, virtual device. As such in a sense it is no different from a conventional clock, in that all clocks use some medium to measure the passing of time: the uncoiling of a spring at a predictable rate, for example, or radioactive decay. Our viral clock depends upon the tendency of viruses to acquire mutations over time. Although viral mutation is a random event, it occurs at a predictable rate. Retroviruses like HIV have a comparatively high rate of mutation. Thus we can plot the moment in time at which the virus deviated from its ancestors to become the species that we now know.

It is now generally accepted that HIV-1 is a mutant version of a chimpanzee virus, SIVcpz. HIV-2, the rarer variant, probably has a similar origin but came from different apes. The virus almost certainly entered circulation among humans through butchery and consumption of meat. There is overwhelming evidence to support this. The genes are highly similar; we know that humans can acquire other retroviruses from butchering apes; it has been demonstrated that the transmission continues in modern times. There is one major obstacle to the hypothesis: SIVcpz appears to cause no illness in apes. This is clearly quite different from the situation among humans.

At some point in history SIV changed to become HIV, in a mutation that allowed the virus to enter human cells and cause disease. Our viral clock, which depends on mutations, allows us to pinpoint this moment with some accuracy. The best available information now suggests that SIVcpz became HIV-1 in the early 20th century. We can also pinpoint where, geographically, that mutation arose. It would appear to have been in West Africa.

There are those who argue that a further, more shameful factor can be entered into the equation. It was first proposed in 2000 by Jim Moore, an American specialist in primate behaviour, who published his findings in the journal *AIDS Research and Human Retroviruses*. At about the time when our viral clock suggests HIV began to cause illness in humans, the exploitation of Africa by western colonialists was at its peak. In some countries such as French Equatorial Africa and the Belgian Congo, labour camps were established with brutally repressive regimes. Hygiene was poor, disease rife and food scarce. There was every incentive for labourers to obtain bush meat to supplement their supplies.

Moore hypothesises that hybridisation of viruses might easily have occurred in such circumstances, and that relatively inert SIV from an infected ape taken as bush meat could have been transmitted to humans already infected with other, unknown viruses. Labourers were permitted access to prostitutes, and rudimentary vaccination with scant regard for sterility of needles may have been carried out. The truth is difficult to confirm because records were systematically destroyed, but both would have provided ready routes of transmission for a blood-borne virus.

This is a convincing, and depressing, possible account of the epicentre of the subsequent pandemic. Deaths in the camps were commonplace; symptoms and signs of a new disease would have passed unnoticed. It should be remembered that this remains a hypothesis, and even if it is correct it does not fully explain how the disease became a global pandemic. Human sexual behaviour and migration had to change to permit this state of affairs. However, it is considerably more convincing than competing theories, such as the one that postulates that the CIA and an organisation called the Special Cancer Virus Program conspired to massacre blacks and gay men.

Moore's hypothesis would be supported if we identified other HIV-infected individuals prior to the first cases appearing in the early 1980s. This has indeed been the case. Most intriguingly the earliest known positive blood sample was taken in 1959 from a man living in what is now the Democratic Republic of Congo. The virus has also been found in tissue samples from an American teenager who died in St Louis in 1969 and from a Norwegian sailor who died around 1976.

The 'new' infections have thus all arisen in man through our greed and curiosity. As such they simply reflect the essence of being human. We could have avoided them all, indeed most infectious disease, simply by not moving from the room in which we were born. Richard did not 'have' to go to Indonesia, in the sense of it being a biological need in the same way that swallows migrate to Africa. He went out of curiosity, and thus put himself at risk of Dengue. You could argue that the pig farmers who exposed themselves to Nipah virus were driven by a biological need – hunger – except that this is not subsistence farming, but for profit.

There could be no better example of this than HIV. If we accept this suggestion of its origins, a simian virus mutating in the starved and already diseased bodies of enslaved Africans in their labour camps, then our rapacity and ruthless curiosity are exposed at their starkest. Should we blame ourselves? Humans are inquisitive, tool-using creatures. A natural consequence of those defining features is that we hunt out new habitats and use those tools to exploit them. We cannot help ourselves. Thus we are epidemics in that exposure to novel infectious diseases is an inevitable consequence of our restlessness, our artifice and our very essence.

The emergence of new epidemics in our recent history leads us to an obvious question. Is there one lurking which could arise to kill every one of us?

CHAPTER 11

CONCLUSION

One of the most memorable statistics I recall from medical school is that enough botulinum toxin to kill the entire population of the world could be stored in a beer can. Saddam Hussein was said at one time to have stored 19,000 litres of it, suggesting he was planning quite a party. Merely 100 grams would be adequate to kill every one of us. Without treatment the consequence would be exactly that: with the possible exception of a few people who had survived a previous attack of botulism from the same strain, all of us would die. In reality it would be impossible to deliver the toxin to every human on the planet simultaneously. Nevertheless the point remains that a naturally occurring substance, a product of common bacteria, is theoretically capable of apocalyptic mortality.

Is it then possible that an epidemic of some other infectious agent might have the same effect? Is there an Armageddon bug out there somewhere, which might immolate every one of us?

Annihilation foreseen

There are a number of conditions that must be met for a true annihilator. First, it should be an entirely new disease, or a variant of an existing one that has mutated sufficiently that humans have not evolved significant immunity to it. This is one of the reasons scientists are so anxious about avian influenza. Once it has made the leap from animals to humans it will effectively be an entirely new virus, for reasons that are explained in Chapter 1. That property persists once the virus has evolved the capacity to transmit from human to human.

A disease that has circulated historically among humans will inevitably have allowed some to develop immunity. There are exceptions to this: effective immunity has never been demonstrated to, for example, HIV, because the virus is so skilled at evading it. There is a separate hereditary resistance to that virus, the CCR5 delta-32 mutation; however, this almost certainly arose as a consequence of some other infection, not HIV.

Our annihilator strain must be readily transmissible and cause sudden, acute illness rather than slowly progressive disease with a long latent period which might allow populations to reproduce and recover. Obviously, it must have a very high case fatality rate. At first sight it may seem more obvious that it should have 100 per cent mortality, but it is possible that this would not be an absolute necessity. The social and political consequences of deaths of even modest proportions of the global population from a single epidemic would be catastrophic.

Imagine an outbreak with a 50 per cent case fatality that affected 20 per cent of the population. Consider the headlines in the newspapers after 6 million deaths in Britain, 26 million in the United States. There would be mass panic, serious threats to law and order, overwhelmed hospitals, chaos. We do not need to imagine such disorder, we have historical records that describe it in considerable detail. Medieval writers such as Boccaccio graphically recount the collapse in social order at the height of the plague years.

Suppose, then, that a disease with less than complete case fatality disrupted the socio-economic stability of even developed nations. Disrupted, chaotic social conditions would then lead to the kind of displaced populations susceptible to further epidemic disease. Serial waves of different epidemics could have the effect that a single infection could not. Further, while it is not likely that an epidemic would kill every single one of us, the certainty of the survival of our 'civilisation' must be far less assured.

Risks high and low

Most of the illnesses we have encountered so far have involved a proportional mortality, even untreated. Avian influenza, the source of one of our chief current anxieties, has a mortality rate in the order of 60 per cent. Even HIV/AIDS, once considered to be uniformly fatal, now appears to be unable to infect a proportion of humanity due to the naturally occurring CCR5 delta-32 mutation. Besides, the population at risk would naturally be restricted to those who had contact with the virus. Nuns, for instance, would be at very low risk of HIV, unless they had been haemophiliacs before proper measures were taken to exclude HIV from pooled blood products, or took the wording of their vows of celibacy extremely liberally.

This also applies to diseases that do appear to lead almost always to death – rabies, for instance. This is a disease that, once it causes symptoms, is lethal in virtually 100 per cent of cases. Rabies is an unlikely annihilator strain, partly because the route of transmission (bites) is readily preventable, and partly because there is a vaccine available both for prevention and for treatment after exposure. In the context of total global chaos, though, rabies could indeed be responsible for the sort of secondary plagues that might sweep nations as packs of feral dogs roamed free.

Ultimate containment of any global pandemic would rely on a number of factors, the earliest being an attempt at physical containment and maintenance of social order. Subsequently treatment and vaccination would be paramount. It is worth noting that of the top ten major pandemics of history identified in the Introduction, there is no truly effective vaccine for almost half. The unpreventable five are typhus, HIV, malaria, tuberculosis and syphilis.

The most real of the potential epidemic threats is influenza, as has already been said. There can be no proper vaccine for the precise strain of avian influenza until the real human disease appears, the one that can be transmitted from person to person. There would be no point in developing a vaccine for the virus that caused the 1918 outbreak, because that was an entirely different strain, H1N1. There is a debate between scientists about how to move forward on a vaccine for the worrying potential modern H5N1 strain. Some feel an imperfect vaccine, raised against the strain that has already killed humans, would be better than nothing. Others take precisely the opposite view, saying that a partially effective vaccine might actually make matters worse, by masking disease yet permitting transmission.

It may not be generally realised, but the H5N1 viruses that have been killing people and animals are far from identical. Those that have arisen in Thailand, Cambodia and Vietnam are different from those in China and Indonesia. Which, if any, should be chosen as the target of a vaccine? There are technical difficulties in developing the vaccine in any event. Because it is a disease of birds, the normal method of developing flu vaccines – injecting the strain into embryonated hens' eggs – does not work, because it kills the embryos. It is also of course extremely hazardous for researchers, and the virus must be handled in rigorously controlled conditions. Attempts to generate a vaccine rely on genetic modification of viral strains – extracting a portion of the gene which will generate immunity with the toxic element removed.

How people and animals behave

The experience of populations exposed to completely new infections can be deduced from historical example, among both humans and animals. We have the example of myxomatosis in rabbits and the plagues listed in the Introduction among humans. Even the most catastrophic – the Black Death and Spanish flu – failed to annihilate humankind, and civilisations did recover. I do not believe there is a naturally occurring bacterium or virus that could kill us all. I stress the word 'naturally'.

The capacity of humans to manipulate microorganisms has moved way beyond science fiction. We are already able to engineer yeasts, for example, to produce human insulin and useful vaccines. There is no reason that some group with evil intent and the right skills could not manipulate a common virus or bacterium to behave quite differently and with extreme malignity. After smallpox was eradicated, laboratory stocks of the virus were destroyed apart from two sites. One is at the Centers for Disease Control in Atlanta, Georgia; the other is in Koltsovo in Siberia. There are rumours that the latter was not safe, and that the virus is already in the hands of the North Koreans and, oddly, the French.

Smallpox had a historical mortality rate of 30 per cent. As the disease has not been encountered for so long and the numbers of the vaccinated have dwindled, nobody knows for certain what the death rate would be if it appeared in the modern era. It could be far worse. Besides, there is no reason that the virus could not be engineered to upgrade its virulence or evade the vaccine. We could take some nervous comfort from the relative failure of modern attempts at bioterrorism. A cult in Japan called Aum Shryinko tried it repeatedly with a broad range of agents, to little effect.

With respect to the most pressing of the modern threats – bird flu – we do actually have treatments as well as those possible if troublesome vaccines, and many governments are urgently stockpiling them. There are essentially three drugs that are active against influenza. The first is amantadine and its derivatives, and the second and third are oseltamivir and zanamavir. Amantadine has been shown to be ineffective against

H5N1. The latter two can treat the disease if given early enough; they work by preventing the virus from being released from cells.

Oseltamivir has been selected as the best agent to control an emerging pandemic, as unlike zanamavir it can be taken by mouth, not inhaled. There has been some suggestion that resistance to oseltamivir has already emerged in Vietnam. That does not automatically mean that the drug would be useless in a pandemic; it just might not work for everyone. The WHO is in the process of amassing millions of doses; currently western stockpiles are in the United States and Switzerland. Roche, the manufacturer, has permitted the production of 'generic' oseltamivir in some countries, notably India and China. A counterfeit drug has already appeared on the market. Treatment for bird flu would probably need to continue for longer than for conventional flu; nobody knows how effective the drug would be during a pandemic and how much resistance would be a problem. There were serious doubts about oseltamivir's efficacy when it was used in Vietnam in 2005, although it may have been prescribed too late.

The drug dearth

We should now look at why so few anti-infective drugs are coming forward. Suppose you are the chief executive officer of a major pharmaceutical company. The heads of two of your research teams come to see you one day, each with a new discovery. One says that he has identified a new compound, which appears safe to use and is active against the bacillus that causes tuberculosis. It is effective against even those growing number of strains that have become resistant to other antibiotics. His colleague then speaks. The other team have developed a slight variant on existing compounds for treating high blood pressure. It is slightly better than the current products, although not much, and has a long list of possible side-effects as well as being expensive to produce. In which do you choose to invest your shareholders' money?

At first sight it seems obvious. Surely it is better to address the emerging threat of resistant tuberculosis with a new drug than add to a formulary already loaded with blood pressure treatments? In fact the choice is not so straightforward. As CEO you have a duty to ensure your shareholders obtain a return on their investment. Tuberculosis is a curable condition. It occurs predominantly in poorer countries. The fact is that your new drug is unlikely to make much money. You choose the high blood pressure treatment.

For many years infectious diseases was known as a Cinderella specialty within hospital medicine. By this I mean that it did not attract funding, the number of consultants dwindled, and the number of doctors in training collapsed. This has now begun to reverse. As diseases of infection begin to threaten us once again, the discipline is once more under the spotlight. The phenomenon applied as much to commercial development of medicines as to training and academic disciplines. In the wake of the apparent disappearance of many infectious diseases, many drug companies that had previously funded research into antibiotics and antivirals channelled their energies into more profitable undertakings.

Conclusion

There is clearly a need for new antibiotics. Resistance is a major problem, as we have discussed. There are numerous reasons for the faltering of big drug companies in the development of new agents. Times are leaner for the pharmaceutical industry. Cutting down on expensive and potentially unproductive research is an obvious cost-cutting step; there is a very high fall-out rate in candidate compounds. Further, antibiotics are unusual in that they tend to have rapidly dwindling returns. If they are successful, they lead to a cure and are thus no longer required (and bought), unlike drugs for, say, heart disease. Resistance inevitably emerges, limiting their usefulness. Drugs that combat resistance will target a smaller number of infections, as there is a trend for physicians to keep them in reserve for the most serious situations; more widespread prescribing will inevitably lead to more widespread resistance. This further squeezes profit margins.

There is another issue to be considered in our increasingly litigious age. Suppose we had not discovered penicillin, but did so today. Nevertheless, this is a drug that is known to cause fatal reactions. Penicillin itself kills between 500 and 1,000 people per year. There is no question that the balance is heavily tilted in favour of benefit rather than risk. Nevertheless, suppose deaths occurred during the trial phase. There is no certainty that the drug would gain a licence nowadays.

The situation is not utterly bleak. Britain's Wellcome Trust has recently awarded £12 million to Prolysis Ltd, a venture capital-backed company based in Oxfordshire, as seed-corn funding to develop next-generation antibacterial drugs against life-threatening, hospital-acquired and community-associated staphylococcal infections. There are others – a company called Cubist has taken up a novel antibiotic called daptomycin which shows promise. Nevertheless the major pharmaceutical companies do seem to be putting anti-infectives on the back burner.

There are those who believe that legislation could be amended and public funds diverted to shift the balance in favour of research into new antibiotics. As Stuart Levy of Tufts University School of Medicine in Boston, Massachusetts said in *Nature* magazine, 'these are societal drugs'. Part of the problem is that sufferers from infections involving resistant organisms are a disparate, widely dispersed group who have little opportunity to exert pressure on governments and pharmaceutical companies. This need not automatically be the case. An example has been set for the world of how concerted, informed, committed and persistent action by the public can achieve results in the management of infectious diseases and the development of new drugs.

The sufferers fight the system

In the early 1980s an article in an academic journal describing a group of young men in Los Angeles who had developed an unusual type of pneumonia proved to be a straw in the wind for a gathering storm. In the early days of the epidemic, PWAs (People With Aids), as they chose to be called, sat meekly in public meetings as the various doctors, nurses, lawyers, insurance experts and social workers debated the nature of the disease and its likely outcome. Gradually a sense of frustration began to emerge among PWAs, who felt patronised and excluded. They began to make demands of the medical profession and society at large; to be at the very least treated without prejudice by both.

Over the following years the objectives, efficacy, stridency and confidence of such pressure groups grew rapidly. From what were effectively self-help groups with little hope of influencing policy and drug development, there arose far more motivated and strident voices. Some, such as the Lavender Hill Mob, began to lobby the Centers for Disease Control in Atlanta to demand more rapid testing and approval for anti-HIV drugs. They identified cumbersome bureaucratic procedures, particularly in clinical drug trials, which slowed the process even as people were dying.

Gradually they decided to politicise their objectives more clearly. An activist called Larry Kramer ended a speech at the Lesbian and Gay Community Services Center in New York's Greenwich Village with the question: 'Do we want to start a new organisation devoted solely to political action?' The answer was a resounding 'Yes!' The question was then asked, what should they do? The response gave the most militant and effective of the pressure groups its title. 'Act up! Fight back! Fight AIDS!' The subsequent meeting of activists came to be known as the AIDS Coalition to Unleash Power, with the acronym ACT UP.

ACT UP developed a slogan, 'Drugs into bodies', which summarised its aims. They were to mobilise funding for development of new drugs, to speed up the torpid and bureaucratic testing process, and to make the drugs affordable. ACT UP felt that time was too short for such scientific niceties as the double-blind trial, which is the gold standard of drug testing. A double-blind trial involves giving one group of subjects a drug and another group a treatment identical in appearance but made of a harmless placebo. It is then possible to compare the two groups to assess the drug; inevitably it means that one group will not be receiving treatment.

There followed a coordinated campaign of headline-grabbing marches, which developed into direct action. Most memorably, ACT UP unfolded the AIDS Memorial Quilt on the National Mall during the second National Lesbian and Gay March on Washington in October 1987. Each panel of the huge quilt represented someone who had died of the disease. A leaflet was handed out to passers-by, which included this message: 'These people have died of a virus. But they have been killed by our government's neglect and inaction ... Before this Quilt grows any larger, turn your grief into anger. TURN THE POWER OF THE QUILT INTO ACTION.'

The ACT UP movement spread, and soon had branches in Sydney, London, Berlin, Amsterdam, Montreal and Paris as well as numerous North American cities. It achieved most through its often strident and aggressive direct actions. These included a brief occupation of the US headquarters of the pharmaceutical company Burroughs-Wellcome, followed by a successful protest directed at the same company on the floor of the New York Stock Exchange, using foghorns and a banner to protest at the price of AZT. The Centers for Disease Control in Atlanta, whose job is to coordinate the US government's response to epidemics, witnessed many actions from the local chapter of

ACT UP. There were many more, and attendees at conferences concerned with AIDS and HIV will recall being heckled and barracked by ACT UP activists.

The effectiveness of these pressure groups in altering the management of their condition has undoubtedly had effects elsewhere in healthcare. Virtually every hospital in Britain, for example, now has a patient advisory and liaison service which seeks to act as advocates for sometimes voiceless individuals who can easily feel intimidated by the system. The balance of power has definitely shifted somewhat. Patients are now regarded as 'health consumers', and they feel able to challenge their physician's advice. Many such groups now exist. The power of such groups to influence policy, and drug testing and development for other infectious diseases, is far less obvious, however.

Tactics and resistance

There is a further point to be made about the pressure groups that demanded 'drugs into bodies'. Resistance in HIV emerges serially. By this I mean that people with the virus can more easily produce mutations that confer resistance to any drug when it is prescribed on its own. The concept that a combination of drugs might prevent this outcome emerged in about 1996. It could be argued that pressure groups demanding early prescribing of single agents brought about a worse outcome for themselves, as their viruses developed resistance to each successive drug.

It is easy to be critical in hindsight, and we can readily understand the urgency of those demands when the death toll was so high. It may also be true that demanding an end to the gold standard of double-blind trials might have muddied the scientific waters. These are carping criticisms, and have to be set against the undoubted efficacy of a group of informed, motivated and politically savvy activists in forcing the pace of drug development. HIV appeared in 1981; really effective treatment (although no cure) became available a mere 15 years later. It is hard to think of any other human illness (with the possible exception of hepatitis C, the treatment of which undoubtedly benefited from research into HIV) that has been tackled so promptly.

There is a final thought about the pressure for HIV treatment and its consequences. Research has been directed largely at drugs active against HIV-1. Some of them are not active at all against HIV-2, the West African variant. The vast majority of research has been directed against HIV-1. Ultimately what is needed is a vaccine that will protect people against both strains of HIV.

We still have no truly effective vaccines for tuberculosis and malaria, two of the major killers in the developing world, and the rate of development of new drugs for these increasingly resistant infections has certainly slowed. Pressure and investment in the West to tackle western diseases have been the story for pharmaceutical development for decades. The world's most profitable and widely prescribed pharmaceutical has been a drug for acid indigestion, barely the most pressing problem given the mortality from infectious disease.

A final note

I hope that this book has demonstrated how much humans are immersed in, formed of and moulded by epidemics. This is something which applies to all of us; we are all the same in the global village. We are epidemics, all of us.

It may also have become obvious throughout this book that our battle with epidemics has been with a relatively small number of microorganisms that cause disease, while the massive majority either do us no harm or are beneficial to us. We may even harness the beneficial power of the microbes for our own benefit.

I shall end on a note of hope. Should the scientific consensus about global warming be correct, and the release of waste gases from human activity into the atmosphere be the cause of the climate change which so threatens us, then these tiny but prolific life forms offer us some hope. Some kinds of marine microbes are capable of 'sinking' atmospheric carbon emissions back into the oceans. The American J Craig Venter Institute has funded a project called the Sorcerer II Expedition, which has been exploring the seas from Canada to the eastern tropical Pacific to hunt for such life-forms, the vast majority of which have not been characterised.

What a delicious turn of events it would be for the purposes of my hypothesis, if this venture discovered a microbe which could save the day for us. We arose from microbes, the microbes made our planet habitable, we are made of microbes, we are moulded by microbes in their epidemic form, we have risked our future by behaving like an epidemic of microbes – and finally we might be saved by them.

FURTHER READING

Traditionally medical and scientific books have bibliographies with numerical references inserted in the text. My experience with such schemes is that they are of little interest to the general reader, and tend rather to interrupt the smooth flow and pleasure of reading. Further, much of the text is derived from personal experience and opinion rather than such facts as may be obtained from textbooks or academic journals. The purpose of this section is to direct the interested reader to further texts and sources rather than to support the claims contained in the book by detailed reference. I have included some journal references where it seemed unavoidable.

Undoubtedly, in my view the best books on infectious diseases are the following. However, they are long, detailed and aimed at practising doctors rather than general readers.

Cook, Gordon and Zumla, Alimuddin (2002) *Manson's Tropical Diseases*, W B Saunders, Oxford

Hoeprich, Paul D (1972) *Infectious Diseases: A guide to the understanding and management of infectious processes*, 1st edn, Harper & Row, New York

Mandell, Gerald L, Bennett, John E and Dolin, Raphael (eds) (2005) *Mandell Douglas and Bennett's Principles and Practice of Infectious Diseases*, 6th edn, Elsevier Churchill Livingstone, Philadelphia, Pa

Introduction

Barry, J M (2004) *The Great Influenza: The epic story of the deadliest plague in history*, Viking, New York

Cartwright, F and Biddiss, M (2004) *Disease and History*, Sutton, Stroud, Glos

Gruzinski, S (1993) *The Conquest of Mexico*, Polity, Cambridge

Huang, Y et al (1996) 'The role of a mutant CCR5 allele in HIV-1 transmission and disease progression', *Nature Medicine*, 2(11) (Nov), pp 1240–43

Margulis, L (2000) *Symbiotic Planet: A new look at evolution*, Basic Books, New York

Oxford, J S et al (2005) 'A hypothesis: the conjunction of soldiers, gas, pigs, ducks, geese and horses in northern France during the Great War provided the conditions for the emergence of the 'Spanish' influenza pandemic of 1918–1919', *Vaccine*, 23(7), pp 940–45

Sass, E J, Gottfried, G and Sorem, A (1996) *Polio's Legacy: An oral history*, University Press of America, Lanham, Md

The Human Genome Project, including an explanation of its aims and achievements, is available on http://www.genome.gov/10001772

Chapter 1

There are texts about viruses aimed at the general reader:

Crawford, Dorothy (2002) *The Invisible Enemy: A natural history of viruses*, pbk edn, Oxford University Press, Oxford

Oldstone, Michael B A (1998) *Viruses, Plagues and History*, Oxford University Press, Australia

The literature on mobile genetic elements is principally within the academic domain at present. The following two books have been written on the subject:

Miller, W J and Capy, P (eds) (2004) *Mobile Genetic Elements: Protocols and genomic applications*, Humana Press, Totowa, NJ

Shapiro, J A (ed) (1983) *Mobile Genetic Elements*, Academic Press, Oxford

These publications are also relevant:

Bellaby, P (2005) 'Has the UK government lost the battle over MMR?', *British Medical Journal*, 330, pp 552–53

Fraenkel-Conrat, H and Williams, R C (1955) 'Reconstitution of active tobacco mosaic virus from its inactive protein and nucleic acid components', *Proceedings of the National Academy of Science* (USA), 41, pp 690–98

Jennings, R and Read, R (2006) *Influenza: Human and avian in practice*, Royal Society of Medicine Press, London

Miller, S (1953) 'A production of amino acids under possible primitive earth conditions', *Science*, 117, pp 528–29

Miller, S and Urey, H (1959) 'Organic compound synthesis on the primitive earth', *Science*, 130, pp 245–51

Chapter 2

Boccaccio, Giovanni (1921) *The Decameron Of Giovanni Boccaccio*, trans J M Rigg, privately published, London

Cook, G C (2001) 'Influence of diarrhoeal disease on military and naval campaigns', *Journal of the Royal Society of Medicine*, 94(2) (Feb), pp 95–7

Dormandy, Thomas (2000) *The White Death: A history of tuberculosis*, New York University Press, New York

Fenner, F and Fantini, B (1999) *Biological Control of Vertebrate Pests: The history of myxomatosis – an experiment in evolution*, CABI, Geneva

Hancock, R E (2001) 'Cationic peptides: effectors in innate immunity and novel antimicrobials', *Lancet Infectious Diseases*, 1(3) (Oct), pp 156–64

Hayes, R A and Richardson, B J (2001) 'Biological control of the rabbit in Australia: lessons not learned?', *Trends in Microbiology*, 9(9) (Sept), pp 459–60

Hirst, L F (1953) *The Conquest of Plague*, Clarendon Press, Oxford

Knell, Robert J (2003) 'Syphilis in Renaissance Europe: rapid evolution of an introduced sexually transmitted disease?', *Royal Society Biology Letters*

McNeill, W (1977) *Plagues and Peoples*, updated edn, Anchor, New York

Von Hutten, U (1519/1945) *A Treatise of the French Disease*, trans in R H Major, *Classic Descriptions of Disease*, 3rd edn, Charles C Thomas, Springfield, Ill

This is an excellent website about Quorum sensing: http://www.nottingham.ac.uk/quorum/

Chapter 3

There are very few texts about parasites for the general reader. A shorter textbook which may be accessible is:

Gillespie, Stephen H and Hawkey, P M (1995) *Medical Parasitology: A practical approach*, Oxford University Press, Oxford

Other references:

Desowitz, Robert S (1993) *The Malaria Capers: More tales of parasites and people – research and reality*, W W Norton, New York

Esch, Gerald W (2007) *Parasites and Infectious Disease: Discovery by serendipity and otherwise*, Cambridge University Press, Cambridge, UK

Chapter 4

Eldridge, B F and Edman, J D (eds) (2003) *Medical Entomology: A textbook on public health and veterinary problems caused by arthropods*, 2nd edn, Springer, New York

Fleischmann, Wim, Grassberger, Martin and Sherman, Ronald (2003) *Maggot Therapy: A handbook of maggot-assisted wound healing*, Thieme, New York

Service, M (2004) *Medical Entomology for Students*, 3rd edn, Cambridge University Press, Cambridge, UK

Yerges, Karen P (2006) *Confronting Lyme Disease: What patient stories teach us*, Booksurge, Charleston, SC

There is an interesting website which includes more information about insects and larvae pressed into medical service at http://biotherapy.md.huji.ac.il/

Chapter 5

Such books as are available for the general reader on the subject of fungi tend to concentrate on edible and psychotropic fungi rather than disease. There is a basic, readable textbook which discusses the structure of fungi and the diseases they cause:

Deacon, Jim (2005) *Fungal Biology*, Blackwell, Oxford

If you absolutely must read about the so-called Candida syndrome, try:

Winderlin, Christine and Sehnert, Keith (1996) *Candida-Related Complex: What your doctor might be missing*, Taylor, Lanham, Md

Other references:

Caporael, Linnda R (1976) 'Ergotism: the Satan loosed in Salem?', *Science*, 192, pp 21–26

Hardin, B D, Kelman, B J and Saxon, A (2003) 'Adverse human health effects associated with molds in the indoor environment', *Journal of Occupational and Environmental Medicine*, 45(5) (May), pp 470–78

True, H L and Lindquist, S L (2000) 'A yeast prion provides a mechanism for genetic variation and phenotypic diversity', *Nature*, 407(6803) (28 Sept), pp 477–83

Chapter 6

Aceh Epidemiology Group (2006) 'Outbreak of tetanus cases following the tsunami in Aceh province, Indonesia', *Global Public Health*, 1(2) (June), pp 173–77

Campanella, N (1999) 'Infectious diseases and natural disasters: the effects of Hurricane Mitch over Villanueva municipal area, Nicaragua', *Public Health Review*, 27(4), pp 311–19

Dunnill, Michael (2000) *The Plato of Praed Street: The life and times of Almroth Wright*, RSM Press, London

Halliday, S (2001) *The Great Stink of London: Sir Joseph Bazalgette and the cleansing of the Victorian metropolis*, Sutton, Stroud, Glos

Morgan, O (2004) 'Infectious disease risks from dead bodies following natural disasters', *Revista Panamericana de Salud Publica*, 15(5), pp 307–12

Sehn, Jan (1957) 'Concentration Camp Oswiecim-Brzezinka (Auschwitz-Birkenau)', translated by Klemens Keplicz, Warszawa, Wydawn

Woodham-Smith, C (1979) *The Great Hunger: Ireland 1845–1849*, Penguin, Harmondsworth

Zinsser, Hans (1984) *Rats, Lice, and History*, reprint edn, Back Bay Books, Boston, Massachusetts

Web references:
http://www.nlm.nih.gov/medlineplus/naturaldisasters.html
Data on mortality from Hurricane Katrina may be found on http://www.cdc.gov/mmwr/preview/mmwrhtml/mm5509a5.htm

Chapter 7

Alm, J S et al (1999) 'Atopy in children of families with anthroposophic lifestyle', *Lancet*, 353 (1 May), p 1485

Bjorksten, B et al (1998) 'Prevalence of childhood asthma, rhinitis and eczema in Scandinavia and Eastern Europe', *European Respiratory Journal*, 12(2) (Aug), pp 432–37

Cooke, A et al (1999) 'Infection with *Schistosoma mansoni* prevents insulin dependent diabetes mellitus in non-obese diabetic mice', *Parasite Immunology*, 21(4), pp 169–76

Correa, P A, Gomez, L M, Cadena, J and Anaya, J M (2005)

'Autoimmunity and tuberculosis: opposite association with TNF polymorphism', *Journal of Rheumatology*, 32(2) (Feb), pp 219–24

Ewald, P W (2000) *Plague Time: How stealth infections cause cancer, heart disease, and other deadly ailments*, Free Press, New York

Lau, S and Matricardi, P (2003) 'Worms, asthma, and the hygiene hypothesis', *Lancet*, 367(9522), pp 1556–58

Marshall, Barry (2002) *Helicobacter Pioneers: Firsthand accounts from the scientists who discovered helicobacters, 1892–1982*, Blackwell Science, Oxford

Summers, R W, Elliott, D E, Urban, J F Jr, Thompson, R and Weinstock, J V (2005) *Trichuris suis* therapy in Crohn's disease, *Gut*, 54, pp 87–90

This article details some information on HERVs in a fairly accessible manner:

Nelson, P N, Carnegie, P R et al (2003) 'Demystified . . . human endogenous retroviruses', *Molecular Pathology*, 56(1) (Feb), pp 11–18

Chapter 8

Alper, T, Cramp, W A, Haig, D A and Clarke, M C (1967) 'Does the agent of scrapie replicate without nucleic acid?', *Nature*, 214, pp 764–66

Alper, T, Haig, D A and Clarke, M C (1966) 'The exceptionally small size of the scrapie agent', *Biochemical and Biophysical Research Communications*, 22, pp 278–84

Battacharya, Shaoni (2003) 'Predicted deaths from vCJD slashed', www.newscientist.com/hottopics/bse/bse.jsp?id=ns 99993440, 26 February (accessed 22 June 2007)

Griffith, J S (1967) 'Self-replication and scrapie', *Nature*, 215, pp 1043–44

Kimberlin, R H (1982) 'Scrapie agent: prions or virinos?', *Nature*, 297, pp 107–08

Manuelidis, L (2004) 'A virus behind the mask of prions?', *Folia Neuropathologica*, 42 Suppl B, pp 10–23

Schwartz, Maxime and Schneider, Edward (2004) *How the Cows Turned Mad: Unlocking the mysteries of mad cow disease*, University of California Press, Berkeley, Calif

Todd, N V et al (2005) 'Cerebroventricular infusion of pentosan polysulphate in human variant Creutzfeldt-Jakob disease', *Journal of Infection*, 50(5) (June), pp 394–96

Van Zwanenberg, P and Millstone, E (2005) *BSE: Risk, science, and governance*, Oxford University Press, Oxford

The website for the CJD surveillance unit in Edinburgh is http://www.cjd.ed.ac.uk/

Chapter 9

This website is very readable:
http://www.niaid.nih.gov/factsheets/antimicro.htm

Das, P (2003) 'Antibiotic resistance in Europe', *Lancet Infectious Diseases*, 3(7) (July), p 398

Reichman, Lee and Tanne, Janice (2000) *Timebomb: The*

global epidemic of multi-drug resistant tuberculosis, Schaum, New York

Salyers, A A and Whitt, D D (2005) *Revenge of the Microbes: How bacterial resistance is undermining the antibiotic miracle*, ASM Press, Washington, DC

Singer, R S et al (2003) 'Antibiotic resistance: the interplay between antibiotic use in animals and human beings', *Lancet Infectious Diseases*, 3(1) (Jan), pp 47–51

There is more about David Livermore, who is the leading UK expert on antibiotic resistance, on http://www.hpa.org.uk/hpa/news/phls_archive/infections_news/2001/010720.htm

Chapter 10

Abraham, T (2005) *Twenty-First Century Plague: The story of SARS*, Johns Hopkins University Press, Baltimore, Md

Chitnis, A, Rawls, D and Moore, J (2000) 'Origin of HIV Type 1 in colonial French Equatorial Africa?', *AIDS Research and Human Retroviruses*, 16(1) (Jan), pp 5–8

Garrett, L (1994) *The Coming Plague: Newly emerging diseases in a world out of balance*, Farrar Straus Giroux, New York

Hooper, E and Hamilton, W (1999) *The River: A journey to the source of HIV and AIDS*, Little, Brown, Boston, Mass

McNeill, John R (2005) 'Yellow fever and globalization', *The Globalist*, Sept, p 70

Wolfe, N D (2004) 'Naturally acquired simian retrovirus infections in central African hunters', *Lancet*, 363(9413) (20 Mar), pp 932–37

Zhu, Tuofu, Korber and Nahinias (1998) 'An African HIV-1 sequence from 1959 and implications for the origin of the epidemic', *Nature*, 391, pp 594–97

The debate about the origins of HIV may also be viewed, with further fascinating material, on http://www.anthro.ucsd.edu/~jmoore/publications/HIVorigin.html

Chapter 11

Alibek, K and Handelman, S (2000) *Biohazard: The chilling true story of the largest covert biological weapons program in the world – told from inside by the man who ran it*, Delta, New York

Hopkins, D R (1983) *Princes and Peasants: Smallpox in history*, Chicago University Press, Chicago

Stuart Levy on the dearth of new anti-infective drugs coming forward can be found on www.nature.com/nsu/030915/030915-6.html

Most of the AIDS activism groups may befound on http://aids.about.com/od/aidsactivism/AIDS_Activism.htm

GLOSSARY

agar A seaweed extract used as a solid medium for culturing bacteria.

allergen A substance which leads to an allergic or 'atopic' response.

amoeba Simple single-celled life form; more complex than bacteria in having a nucleus and an outer membrane.

antigenic drift The method by which the influenza virus changes slightly to cause smaller, localised outbreaks.

antigenic shift The method by which the influenza virus suddenly and dramatically changes to become more dangerous and potentially cause global pandemics.

AZT (Azidothymidine) A failed cancer drug which became the first effective treatment for HIV.

balanced polymorphism The inheritance of disease characteristics as a trade-off for resistance to infection.

biofilms A community of varied microbes – bacteria, fungi, algae – which sticks to surfaces. Within the community there is sharing, communication and cooperation between species.

black building syndrome The supposed illness that arises from living in a building contaminated with certain moulds.

BSE (bovine spongiform encephalopathy) Mad Cow Disease.

candida A common yeast, with many species, which may cause vulvo-vaginal candidiasis.

cationic antimicrobial peptides Another name for defensins.

chloroplasts The plant equivalent of mitochondria.

chromosome A collection of genes and some proteins arranged in functional units. Humans have 23 pairs. Bacteria have a single one.

cytokines Protein chemicals released by immune cells which change the activity of their neighbours to coordinate the collective response.

defensins Substances naturally produced in body fluids which are capable of killing microbes.

DIC (disseminated intravascular coagulation) The final, usually fatal consequence of a number of diseases where the blood ceases to clot properly and death is by bleeding. Infections are a common, if not the sole, cause.

DNA (deoxyribose nucleic acid) The chemical which composes the genes of most life forms.

DNA helix The structure of DNA is famously arranged in a spiral, helical form.

Ebola A rare but often lethal viral infection mostly confined to Africa. Death is by haemorrhage.

endocrine Concerning the method of production and the effects of hormones.

enteroviruses Group of viruses which reproduces in the intestine, although rarely causing disease there.

enzymes Proteins which do the work of transforming material within living organisms to make them more useful. Really they are catalysts.

eosinophils White blood cells so-called because they absorb a stain called eosin, they have a vital function in immunity to parasites. They are also implicated in asthma and allergy.

ergotism Poisoning with the chemical ergot, which is derived from various plants and moulds.

ERVs (endogenous retroviruses) Viral genetic material found in the genes of animals and passed from parent to offspring. Until recently they were generally considered non-functional, but there is now considerable interest in their role in health and disease. In humans they are known as HERVs (see below).

flavivirus A family of viruses including those which cause yellow fever and hepatitis C.

flora Literally 'plants', in this context it refers to the types of microbes which thrive, usually harmlessly, in a given site.

formulary List of drugs available within a hospital or medical practice.

gene An hereditary unit, composed of DNA which determines, via a code, the characteristics of the life-form.

HERVs (human endogenous retroviruses) A group of retroviruses which has become permanently incorporated into human chromosomes.

HIV (human immunodeficiency virus) The agent of AIDS.

HIV/AIDS AIDS is the acquired immunodeficiency syndrome, which results when HIV has killed enough white blood cells to damage immunity.

hormones Chemical messengers like insulin which circulate around the body and have their effects distant from their site of production.

Human Genome Project Completed in 2003, a 13-year project coordinated by the US Department of Energy and the National Institutes of Health to identify all the approximately 20,000–25,000 genes in human DNA.

integron A 'gene capture system'. A method by which bacteria may transmit and receive DNA between one another; more complex than plasmids because they are more precise and directed in their actions.

leishmaniasis A parasitic infectious disease of varying severity ranging from skin ulcers to gross facial disfigurement, liver disease and death. A zoonosis.

malaria A parasitic disease transmitted to humans via the bite of a mosquito.

MDR-TB (multi-drug resistant tuberculosis) A worrying variant of one of the world's biggest killers which now no longer responds to two or more antibiotics.

MDT (maggot debridement therapy) The use of maggots to eat diseased flesh.

ME (myalgic encephalomyopathy aka chronic fatigue syndrome) A condition principally defined by tiredness and weakness which some believe may be an abnormal response to a mild infection.

megafauna Pseudo-scientific term for larger animal.

meme The gene of ideas. A unit of information which behaves like a gene and transmits between people.

mitochondrion (*pl* -a) A structure found within the cells of many life forms including humans, which produces energy. It was once a bacterium.

MMTV (mouse mammary tumour virus) An ERV that occurs in mice and causes cancer in that animal.

molecule A collection of atoms bound together; they may be of varying complexity.

mutagenesis Formation or development of a mutation, or genetic alteration.

mutagenic See mutagenesis above.

mycotoxins Poisons produced by fungi.

pathogenic Capable of causing disease.

pathogeniticity islands A sequence of DNA that contains genes that code for pathogenic properties. May transmit between bacteria.

picornavirus Another family of viruses including the agent of polio.

plaques Ribose nucleic acid. Some viruses have this as their genes instead of DNA. It is also used by many life forms as an intermediary in making proteins and in reproduction.

plasmid A unit of DNA found in bacteria separate from its chromosome which may transmit from one bacterium to another, carrying genes with it.

probiotic flora Flora may be altered to a more healthy mix by adding large quantities of harmless organisms. This is 'probiotics'.

prophylaxis Prevention by medical or artificial methods.

proteases Enzymes which destroy proteins.

protein envelope In this context, the outer casing of a virus, made of protein, which is protective and contains the binding mechanism by which the virus can attach to its victim.

protozoon The group of life forms to which amoebae and malaria belong, being single-celled with a nucleus and an outer membrane.

quorum sensing A method by which bacteria may communicate using chemical signals.

regional strain The sub-type of influenza virus common in a specific location.

retrotransposons Almost the same as transposons, except that they require an added step using RNA.

retroviruses A group of viruses including HIV which are defined by having RNA as their genes and containing the enzyme reverse transcriptase.

ribosomes Cell sub-unit where proteins are produced, a vital function for all cells.

RNA (ribose nucleic acid) Some viruses have this as their genes instead of DNA. It is also used by many life forms as an intermediary in making proteins and in reproduction.

SARS (severe acute respiratory syndrome) A viral illness of the lungs which caused an outbreak of illness in many countries in 2002–03 and killed about 800 people.

sialic acid residues Naturally occurring substance on the surface of cells which forms the site where the influenza virus binds and enters.

SIV (simian immunodeficiency virus) The variant of HIV

which affects some apes. It is believed to have been the origin of human disease.

steroids A group of chemicals of related structure with many different hormone-like functions. Includes sex hormones like testosterone and oestrogen.

streptococci Widespread genus of bacteria, some of which cause disease.

toxin Poison.

TMV (Tobacco Mosaic Virus) The first ever virus to be shown to be infectious, causing discolouration of tobacco plants.

TSEs (transmissible spongiform encephalopathies) The group of diseases to which vCJD and BSE belong.

transposons Sequences of DNA that can move around to different positions within the life form or even between life forms. Also known as 'jumping genes'.

vCJD (variant Creutzfeldt-Jakob disease) A universally fatal brain disease believed to be transmitted to humans by eating contaminated beef. Variant as distinct from the inherited form.

vector A means of transmitting a disease from one victim to another. Often, but not always, an animal.

virulence factor Substance produced by a bacterium which actually causes the disease.

VRE (vancomycin resistant enterococcus) A bacterium of the species Enterococci which has lost its susceptibility to the antibiotic vancomycin. A major problem in many hospitals.

vulvo-vaginal candidiasis Infection and symptoms of the female genital area with yeasts such as candida. Aka thrush.

zoonoses Diseases transmitted to humans from animals.

INDEX

ABOUT THE AUTHOR

Dr Robert Baker trained in London as a consultant in microbiology at King's College Hospital and in infectious diseases at the Royal Free Hospital. He has written many columns and articles and is the author of Atlas of Differential Diagnosis in HIV.